ADD

AND CREATIVITY

Lynn Weiss, Ph.D.

TAYLOR PUBLISHING COMPANY
DALLAS, TEXAS

Published by Taylor Publishing Company
1550 West Mockingbird Lane
Dallas, Texas 75235

Book design by Mark McGarry
Set in Electra

Library of Congress Cataloging-in-Publication Data
Weiss, Lynn
     A.D.D. and creativity : tapping your inner muse / Lynn Weiss.
          p. cm.
     Includes index.
     ISBN 0–87833–960–4 (pbk.)
     1. Attention-deficit disorder in adults—Popular works.   2. Creative ability.
I. Title.
RC394.A85W443   1997
616.85'89—dc21   97–18633
                                                                          CIP

Printed in the United States of America
10 9 8 7 6 5 4 3 2 1

CONTENTS

ACKNOWLEDGMENTS

My heartfelt thanks to all who helped me find my inner voice—the one that speaks from my creative center. It taught me much of what I have been able to share in this book.

Special thanks to my creative support network including:

Jerell Lambert, my composition teacher,

My sons, Aaron and Mendel Weiss, who continue
to believe in me as a person,

My agent, Mary Kelly,

My editors, Janis Dworkis, Holly McGuire, and Mary Schafer,

And Mike Stromberg, the cover artist who captured the
essence of this so nicely in pictorial form.

Additional thanks to all of the people who work at Taylor Publishing Company to make this book's publication and distribution possible.

Final gratitude to the many people who are ADD and who have shared their stories. As they have told their stories to me, I, in turn, have seen the great wealth of creativity that resides within each. The expression of formidable talents living within ordinary people are what A.D.D. and Creativity is all about.

chapter one

Why I Wrote This Book

I F I HAVE the desire to create, does that mean I have talent? With a lump in my throat and tears running down my face, I wrote this question at the top of my journal page in 1988. It's hard to know which was worse that day: the grief that caused the lump in my throat, or the molasseslike confusion that filled my head.

Although still intent on living the professional life I'd led for thirty years, I had been sneaking writing, painting, sculpture, and creative thinking in whenever I could wangle a little time. I felt like a thief skulking around in dark alleys late at night. I hid many of my productions in file cabinets, unable to throw them away but equally unable to bring them out into the light.

Occasionally, I'd find someone with whom I thought it would be safe to share one of my illicit productions. With lowered voice and trembling heart, I'd murmur, "Would you please take a look at this?"

Then my head would start to roar with contradictory messages and desires. One voice would say, *Soon I'll be discovered — a great new playwright, painter, or poet. People will tell the story over and over about how this previously unknown woman and her work were found in the jungles of the city, brought to light by whoever it was I'd picked that day to be exposed to my work.* I could hear the Oohs and Aahs.

But I also heard a countering voice that said, *She'll think I'm foolish. She won't want to be my friend anymore, because she'll think I've been presumptuous.*

Then the litany of painful memories would begin. There was the time I had painted a picture for my mother for Christmas. I'd done it in oils and had worked for many days to get the colors and tones just right. Unwrapping it after a couple of glasses of wine, she'd laughed, pushed it away and said in a nonappreciative voice, "What is this thing?" I was ten then and never painted for her again.

Then there were the lessons I tried to take in art, music, and writing. I never really did very well. I didn't seem to be able to do things the "right" way. My work was never complimented. It never won awards. And the classes always seemed difficult. Yet, on my own, I wrote, painted, sculpted, and constructed projects constantly throughout my life.

But always the question ran through my head, *Am I talented? Am I creative?*

Even in my professional life I saw things differently than the way I had been taught. Ideas would pop into my head spontaneously, based on my experiences, not on what I had read in a text book. For example, based on my work with preschoolers, I developed a theory of human behavior called the Core Components of Human Nature. Later, I began to apply those concepts in my work as a counselor for adults. Effortlessly, my whole approach to counseling and teaching changed as I applied what I knew, the theory that had simply come into my mind.

Yet external recognition, which would have validated the worth of my many "productions," failed to come. No one thought I was particularly bright or smart, much less creative. And what I wanted to be seen as, more than anything else in the world, was creative.

I remember a time when I was a talk-radio host. The question of the day being asked by the host of the show immediately before mine was, What do you want written on your tombstone? What do you most want to be remembered for? Without a moment's hesitation, I said, "Here lies a creative person." The instant I'd heard the question, a visual image of a tombstone had appeared in my mind. And written on it was the coveted phrase.

That's how my mind has always worked. Though I am not a visual learner in relation to the world around me, my mind has nevertheless always held a stage with a play or movie constantly playing. When I'm thinking about a particular question, I "see" the answer played out on the inner screen of my mind. And the plays that I watch on that screen reflect what I feel. I automatically categorize every experience—visual, auditory, kinesthetic, mental, emotional, and spiritual—in terms of how I feel in relation to that particular experience.

That's just what happens inside of me. I never meant it to happen. I don't mind it happening. It's just me.

Over the years, my intellect has tried to sort out all of the things that happened to me relative to creativity, from my mother's inability to appreciate my gift when

I was ten to my continuing desire to be creative. I've needed to understand all of this so I could feel at peace. I also hoped to find the key to fulfill my most deeply held desires.

Several years after writing the poignant question, "If I have the desire to create, does that mean I have talent?" I went back to that same piece of paper and wrote a simple answer—Yes.

The answer came only after I'd learned to validate my own work, irrespective of what outside sources thought or how they responded. My toughest audience proved to be myself. I needed to discover myself—and I did. As I wrote in the last lines of a poem I recently penned for a performing arts production at the Hyde Park Theater in Austin, Texas,

> *I am all that I dreamed and hoped for, you bet,*
> *Now that I'm older, I see,*
> *I can be what I like*
> *Pleasing only myself*
> *In command of my life out and in.*
> *Because I am whole*
> *After all of these years*
> *The fairies and angels return.*
> *I play with the little ones*
> *Under the trees*
> *And fly with the winged ones on high.*
> *For now I am grown and happy with me.*
> *Don't you know!*
> *DON'T YOU KNOW!*

In addition to my lifelong inner desire to express my creativity, I have one other issue that has been with me from birth. And that is the fact that I am ADD—Attention Deficit Disorder. ADD is not really a disorder at all, although that is how it has been labeled by the health-care community. In reality it is simply a particular style of brain wiring—one that seems to go hand in hand with exceptional creativity. As I have learned over time about ADD—my own, my son's, and that of all the people who had shared their lives with me in my role as a counselor—I have come face to face with more creativity per square inch than I had ever dreamed possible. I have never seen a more creative bunch of people.

I realize that the effects of having a creative spirit need to be sorted out from the effects of ADD. And I know that many others, like myself, have struggled, and are still struggling, to figure out how to live life with both ADD and creativity. In particular I am aware of the struggle to deal with sensitivity—an attribute of both ADD and creativity, and one of the most difficult to manage.

I've seen that creativity and ADD can cause enormous amounts of pain, but I don't believe it has to be that way. I don't believe that pain is necessary for growth or to make gains of any kind. I fully know from experience that pain can be eliminated, and healing and growth can gently take its place with results that are enduring.

I've learned a lot about my own creativity and my ADD. I've had hundreds of people share their stories with me about both. I've seen our common struggles. And I've come to realize that the question for us is not, How can I increase my creativity or get creative? but, How can I live with my creativity?

LIVING YOUR DREAM

I am writing this book because I want to share with you all that I've learned about creativity and the ways in which it interacts with ADD. I want you to know that, *If you can dream it, you can do it.* You can be the person you want to be. You wouldn't have such a strong desire if you didn't already have the potential. You are simply recognizing something that belongs to you.

To be sure, the form that your dreams take may vary over time. But you will find a way, if you persevere, to reach those dreams. No one and nothing can stop you permanently. We all get derailed on our journey from time to time, and that can deplete our hopes temporarily. But eventually, you will be able to use every scrap of your experience—even those experiences that seemed negative when they occurred—for the ultimate creation, your life.

Creativity is a core part of living. It's fundamental. None of us can squelch our creativity without feeling less than whole, incomplete, and depressed. I want to help you reach your wholeness, your feelings of completeness, and your happiness. *I* know you can do it. But *you* are the one who must come to believe it. I believe in you, and I can share that belief with you. But you must take over the job of forming self-belief.

I'm also writing this book because I don't want you to get discouraged. I know how easy it is to get discouraged. And I know that trying to make your ADD style of brain wiring mesh with the demands of a non-ADD culture can sometimes become very discouraging.

I don't want you to become discouraged because giving up on something as important as your creativity is like saying you're not going to breathe anymore because you can't find the air quality you want. It goes against your very nature. Do something to preserve your creativity and yourself, even if it means hiding your creative desires temporarily. Then do something to improve the quality of the polluted air so you can freely enjoy the breath of life.

Do something to nurture yourself. Be with a friend who understands your creative desires. Go on vacation. Do something that will give you joy. Then when you feel re-energized, go about the job of finding a new or different way of exercising your creativity.

That's what I've had to do—many times. For example, twenty-six years ago an animated cartoon played itself out in my mind. I put down on paper what I had seen in my mind. But when I tried to find an animator to work on the cartoon with me, I ran into a lot of roadblocks. So I put the project away for awhile. Ten years ago I pulled my beloved characters out of their file folder and wrote a story to go with the drawings. But again, I couldn't figure out how to get the cartoon produced. Three months ago I talked with a musician who encouraged me to go back to the cartoon. And one month ago I met a man who has a computer-based business with animators on his staff. Now I'm working on the storyboard and script with renewed excitement.

I promise you I will continue to pursue this project to its completion. Twenty-six years after it came to me, I still like this cartoon, believe in it and know there is a role for it in the world.

There are other projects that I've set aside along the way for one reason or another. And I've done that purposely. I continue to support projects that I believe in and see a use for, even if they seem to be at a standstill. That doesn't mean that I don't get discouraged at times. But when that happens, I've learned to back off for awhile, take care of myself and watch for future opportunities. They do come.

All of us humans share common feelings. Sometimes you may feel like you're the only one in the world who is running into creative obstacles. But I promise you that everyone has difficulties along the way just like you do. Sooner or later, however, you will find a new lead that puts you back on track.

The only people who fail are those who quit. Now there's nothing wrong with quitting if you're no longer interested in your creative endeavor or decide that the time has past for it to be useful to others. But don't ever quit just because you're afraid you won't succeed.

I'm writing this book because I want you to honor your creative nature and learn how to manage it to your advantage. That means having some perspective on yourself and the way you're wired, on your desires and how to get them harnessed, and on the necessary practical steps that will lead toward fulfillment. I want you to really appreciate, respect, and free your creativity. I want you to be able to answer the questions, What do I do with all this creativity? What do I do with all my creative energy?

Chances are you've asked yourself those questions many times. Many people with ADD feel so much creative energy bottled up inside that they hardly know what to do with it all. But I'm going to help you learn to direct and express that energy, so you will be able to use your creativity productively.

Our world needs to have creativity reintroduced into daily living. We need creative solutions to solve some of our chronic problems and to balance a world filled with numbers and technology. We need people to work together on heartfelt projects to come up with those creative solutions. After all, when people come together creatively, without competition and one-upmanship, the likelihood of violence and struggle is reduced. That's because creativity brings such joyfulness that it makes it impossible for energy to be spent on hurting others. Instead energy is used to build new and wonderful outcomes that can make the world a better place.

People with ADD have a lot of creativity and can be a strong force for good in the world. Perhaps people who are ADD will be the forerunners who transform our world, changing it for the better. Our numbers are great, and our influence can be powerful.

Once people with ADD can form a positive relationship with their creativity, they can carry the results of that relationship out into the world as a positive force.

My final goal in writing this book is to broaden the definition of creativity to include not just specific talents, but to embrace a creative style of living that is available to many people. By considering this broader definition, you will come to recognize the creativity within yourself and others. Also, as we adults get in touch with our creativity, we will be able to recognize it in our children, cherishing and protecting it. Together we can make our social attitudes and the institutions within which we function, more humane and positive, creating an atmosphere that engenders growth, not conformity.

LOOKING BACK

I believe everyone is born creative. We have an innate drive to open ourselves up in a safe environment, to absorb the stimulation that is ever present around us. As we take in experiences of all kinds, our unique identities are molded and shaped into what will become our special style of living. For those of us with ADD, the attributes and difficulties of ADD greatly influence that style. To the degree that we are supported and surrounded by a healthty environment, we can retain our openness and express our uniqueness in everything we do.

During our preschool years we build feelings of competence and power, the ability to be in charge of ourselves and our expressions. By age six our emotional development culminates in the creation of a value system that, we hope, fits the uniqueness of our creativity and identity. With healthy outside influences that are supportive to our uniqueness, we establish a balance that keeps our creative channels open.

Sometimes, though, the people around us don't know how to create growth-producing environments that honor our individuality. When this happens, our creativity and our expression of it become compromised.

That's what happened to me. And I imagine that might be what happened to you.

Though I have few memories before the age of ten, my most pleasurable memory relates to a creative experience. That's when I felt most alive and in touch with the real me.

I recall going downstairs to my landlady's kitchen table several times when I was about five years old. The landlady, who was previously a kindergarten teacher, presented me with all kinds of circular-shaped objects: large and small plates, glasses of different sizes, jar lids, coins, and cups. She brought out a wonderful box of crayons that had more colors than I had ever seen, and told me I could trace around the circles then color them in. She also showed me how to trace parts of circles to make other geometric figures.

I will never forget how wonderful I felt working with those shapes and colors. Time stood still, and I hated it when I had to leave. I never left that table voluntarily. Throughout my childhood I painted and drew. It was my artwork that kept me alive. I loved colors and shapes and used them to create pictures and picture stories. I've never stopped doing that to this day.

I am told that when I was very young I danced a lot, all around the house. I can remember dancing for my parents and some of their friends, and it's a memory that makes me feel happy. It's as if I can hear some far-off music that propels my body through space. I like the way that makes me feel. Even now, I dance naturally and easily for myself or with others who also like to move their bodies gracefully and rhythmically.

My parents saw my enjoyment in dance and decided to give me dance lessons. But, in contrast to my wonderful memories of dancing around the house, when I recall the dance lessons the only feeling I remember is fear. I remember a constant fear that I wouldn't get the steps right, so I stopped dancing. I must have been about four years old.

My parents gave me piano lessons for a couple of years starting when I was about five or six years old, and those lessons bring much the same fear to mind. I remember being afraid that my music teacher would disapprove of my playing. I sat in terror, fearing I would make a mistake. I remember feeling guilty about

7

the fact that I didn't practice very long each day. I wanted to practice, but because of my ADD, I just couldn't sit still long enough to do it.

For years, though, I played the piano for myself. During my teen years, I developed a moderate level of proficiency. I also wanted to play the flute and drums, but my dad's best friend in college played the saxophone, and my dad wanted me to play it, too. So I did.

I hated playing the saxophone. But I played for seven years because I was afraid to tell my dad how I felt. Consequently, I have a particularly sharp memory of trading instruments with the flute player in the band. I also secretly bought a pair of drum sticks and set up a board in my bedroom to use as a drum. Now I'm not sure how in the world I could have done that secretly, but I felt like I had to hide what I was doing. After all, that was what I really wanted to do, so it had to be wrong. That feeling—the assumption that what I really wanted in my heart was wrong—is one I have experienced many times throughout my life.

In junior high school I had an opportunity to conduct the band. I loved it. In fact, I loved it so much that I was afraid to show my feelings about it. Though I couldn't hear pitch well, I felt the blending of the various instruments and experienced the overall flow of what I wanted the band to produce. Now, forty-five years later, I am enjoying the same creative role of pulling a production together. This time, it's in the performing arts area, combining music, dance, drama, and my writings.

I remember daydreaming a lot as a child. Images, colors, and sounds would float through my mind. When I was about eleven, I saw Walt Disney's *Fantasia*. I was ecstatic! The shapes, colors, and imaginary animals on the movie screen were the same images that had been playing in my mind for as long as I could remember. Seeing that movie gave me hope—hope that somewhere in the world other people like me existed. I didn't quite conceptualize it that way at eleven, but that was the feeling, the feeling of hopefulness.

The first time I ever remember feeling hopeful about my creative desires was just the year before I saw *Fantasia*. That was the day I learned about the planets in science class. The solar system was displayed on a wonderful chart in vivid colors with circles and ellipses spinning in beautiful patterns all across the wall of my schoolroom. After school that day I sat on the steps in front of my home and looked up at the sky. I felt my heart move. And I knew there was something more out there than the world I had known until that time.

Circles, music, planets, and *Fantasia* were the lifelines to my future, and unbeknownst to me, they were integral to the very core of my identity. I just didn't realize it then.

WHAT WENT WRONG

Many things happened in my childhood that turned off my creative juices. But perhaps the most unfortunate is that in the name of *learning*, I could not be creative. From my youngest years the formal educational process allowed me little opportunity to use my hands-on, exploratory, creative strengths for learning purposes. Although those of us with ADD learn best through a hands-on, exploratory approach, my childhood experiences taught me that I should not be creative, and I should not depend on my inner senses to give me solutions. The very process of traditional education guided me away from what was really my strongest teacher—my intuitive, inner guide.

Nevertheless, I did have a few opportunities to soar creatively in childhood. Maybe it's because there were so few of those opportunities that I remember them so vividly.

For example, I remember clearly my fifth-grade language-arts teacher. Reading was hard for me, and I now know that I am dyslexic. Consequently, I had to spend a lot of time struggling to learn information that others breezed through. My teacher, who seemed to recognize that I needed some extra help, began to read aloud to me. And that opened the whole new world of language arts. I remember being very excited about it. But two months later, my family moved away from that school. And I never again experienced the joy of being read to.

That wonderful fifth-grade teacher also encouraged me to write poetry and short stories, which I enjoyed. But once I left her class, I never wrote again for pleasure as a child. My new language-arts teacher seemed to have a never-ending emphasis on punctuation, parts of speech, and diagramming of sentences. Does anyone really know what a past participle is? I haven't a clue to this day. None of those endless exercises helped me learn to write at all, neither as a child nor as an adult.

With writing made into a chore, I only wrote what was required of me—and I didn't do that particularly well. As an adult, I began to keep a secret journal, and that became the vehicle for my eventual emergence as a writer. But I didn't write well until after I had worked as a talk-radio host for some time, and someone suggested that I write the way I speak. That someone was a very special teacher who became my first real book editor and, later, agent.

Ironically, I didn't learn to enjoy reading until after I had begun to write. As my writing began to improve, I began to read spontaneously. Unfortunately, I was in my fifties before this comfort with language arts returned.

Even my art work went underground in school. I recall taking one art class in high school. At the time, I was taking classes in chemistry, analytical geometry, and other subjects that I did not enjoy, so I was very excited about the prospect of art class. But then I discovered that I wasn't good at fashion design and I couldn't draw people realistically. The exercises we were required to do in class were very boring to me, and I became discouraged. I also felt ashamed of my work, although I loved it. Like many people with ADD, I needed excitement, stimulation and validation to keep my interest. I didn't get those, so that was the end of my interest in art class.

I still have a couple of drawings that I made in my high school years when I was allowed to do what I wanted. The teacher didn't think they were great but I think they are some of the best work I have ever produced. They are a vivid, multicolored, fanciful tree with a snake wrapped around its trunk, a country scene with blue and orange trees, and an ad for Ivory soap that featured a swan with bubbles cascading from its back into infinity. I love these drawings. I keep them even now, though the paper has turned a bit yellow with age.

Based on my experiences in that high school art class, I figured that I probably wasn't nearly as creative as I had thought I was. I certainly wasn't talented like my classmates who could draw realistically.

For many reasons, including the fact that I had to work so hard to keep up in school because of my ADD, I had to stuff my creativity deep down inside. Granted, I still used my creativity in secret—dreaming up stories and improvising a drum set. But having to be secretive about my creativity as a child brought on feelings of guilt, guilt that surfaced for many, many years whenever I expressed myself creatively.

The Effects of Parents

One of my long-term secrets was that I wanted to major in one of the creative arts in college. One day, as a high school senior, I found the courage to mention that to my parents. My father immediately assured me that I could never make a living with any of the arts and said I should become a professional. So, feeling guilty for wanting something so irresponsible, I did exactly what he told me to do.

My parents were not bad people. They just did not understand how I learned or what I needed. They held a culturally accepted model of learning that I also embraced because I didn't know any better. Unfortunately, I didn't realize until decades later that that model had little to do with the way in which I, and most people with ADD, learn.

I think my parents genuinely tried to support my creativity by giving me lessons. They never intruded, never told me to stop when I was painting or playing music or just thinking. But neither did they encourage me to talk with them about what I was doing. They never really seemed to appreciate my creative endeavors. And they certainly never encouraged me to pursue them in depth.

I realize now that some of my parents' own emotional needs got in the way of their ability to support my creativity. I feared my father's criticism, though, ironically, he didn't criticize my productions. Rather, he criticized anyone who did art by referring to artists as, "Those punks who waste their time." I was bright enough to understand that if I spent my time hanging out with "punks," I'd be seen as one, too. I wasn't strong enough then to stand up to that kind of criticism on my own two feet.

My mother was so frightened by life in general, so anxious, that she had no time to indulge in the development of her creativity or appreciate mine. I think she had a great deal of creativity, although it never evolved beyond limited needlework and interior decoration. She lacked the confidence to take her lovely work beyond the door of her own home. In another day and time, with confidence, she could have become an interior decorator or artisan. She had the talent, but she didn't have any belief in herself.

As a Result

Graduating from college led me to the workplace, for which I was totally unsuited. But I pounded the pavement, and I managed to get a civil service job in Arizona working with unemployment claims. I hated it. When my six-month probation was up, I asked for a transfer to the employment service. I wanted to work only half time, so that I could spend the rest of my time doing art work.

And that's what I did. For four years I designed and produced silk-screened stationery, place mats and various other small items for sale. I also learned to do some stone carving and ceramic sculpture. But I was shy and afraid to try to market the items I made. Actually, I didn't have a clue as to how to sell, market, or distribute my work. I just wanted to design and develop the pretty pictures in my head.

Going nowhere and making very little money, I moved to New York City on the advice of an older friend who took me under her wing. I told people I was going to study sculpture. But somewhere inside I knew that was not the direction for me. And I was right. I had neither the temperament to be a full-time artist, nor did I do the type of art that could make me a living. I also longed to help other people.

Soon I met a psychotherapist who encouraged me to go to graduate school. He said I was a natural therapist and a sensitive, creative person who would do well helping people. He was involved in the Jungian psychology movement, which respects and utilizes the arts in a more extensive way than most therapies. I resonated to his suggested combination of psychology and the arts, so I went to graduate school.

Over the next three decades I applied my creative skills to mental-health work. I found that the same mind that created pictures in my head also created new and different ways to look at human behavior. I liked following the lead of my inner senses and was able to birth both a theory of human behavior—now called the Core Components of Human Nature—and many books, articles, and programs that helped children and adults get in touch with their identity and the beauty of living. In particular I was able to help many people come to terms with their ADD and learn to see the many ways in which it enriched their lives, as well as find solutions for some of the ways in which it made their lives more difficult.

I felt good about my work. But as the years rolled by, I also felt pain because I lost touch with so much of my artistic creativity. There just wasn't time to make a living as a psychotherapist and talk-show host, raise a family, take care of all the details that city living requires, and pursue creative endeavors.

Of course, looking back, I also realize I wasn't ready to take a stand to honor my creativity. I wasn't emotionally strong enough. I didn't believe in myself enough. I didn't know how to get my work beyond the first step of creation myself, nor how to network with others to help me.

So even though I looked like such a success to the outside world, inside I suffered—worrying that my creativity was withering away and fearing that many of my creations would end up as stillbirths, trapped in the folders of my file cabinet.

Hope for the Future

Nature has a wonderful way of knocking us on the side of the head when we endlessly continue to do things that aren't good for us. My "knock" came when I both burned out as a mental-health professional and was fired from my radio job within a twelve-month period. It took several years to recover from that burn-out and to emerge with a new life. But during those years I learned a lot.

I learned to listen to my heart—and when I listened carefully, I found a part of me that had been locked away for a long time—my creative self. I allowed myself the luxury of spending a lot of time writing in my journal. I found that my feelings wrote themselves in the form of poetry and short stories.

I learned that none of my interest in creativity nor my own creative talents had been permanently lost. In fact I found that my specific skills emerged at a higher level than when I had packed them away years earlier. I knew that my intense desire to create could no longer be ignored. I came to know the meaning of creative passion.

I discovered that a lot of the pain I had suppressed for years was rising up and forcing me to pay attention to its cause. As a result I noticed that I had a strong desire to create in all sorts of media. I wanted to write, make music, draw, paint, and design multimedia works. Most especially, I wanted to do performing arts. I wanted to replicate the stage that existed in my mind and turn it into a real-life stage with dance, music, lighting, and narrative drama.

I also wanted to finish some long-shelved projects. These included animation, teaching books, stories, and books of poetry. I also found a desire to share my experiences so that others could benefit.

I had never really had a teacher or mentor, so I wondered how I was going to accomplish all this. Then one day I symbolically stamped my foot on the ground and said, Okay, Universe. I don't know how I can accomplish any of this, but I have to be able to create, and I have to create well by my standards. I must capture the essence of what is in my mind and heart.

As a result of this invocation the first real teacher of my life came along. I asked her to help me, and she said she would. She taught me to write in a manner that I could grasp—kinesthetically—using methods that my ADD allowed me to pick up quickly. In some ways it was almost as if we wrote together. She would edit my work and explain why changes were necessary. She helped me to simplify my work and she showed me a process of writing that I could follow.

This teacher gave me hope that I could gain some control over my writing, so that I could reflect the richness I felt inside. Slowly hope replaced pain. I found they couldn't exist in the same space.

At the same time, I knew that I had to make a move out of the city into an environment that fit me better. I'd been wanting to make such a move for years. In 1987, I had a dream of a place that I had never seen but a place that was already familiar to me. It was a cliff, and I felt I belonged there. I began to look for it. But it wasn't until the time of my burn-out, when I'd given up on finding it, that a circuitous set of circumstances led me to Central Texas one day.

I'm sure you can guess what I saw when I looked up at a For Sale sign perched on some land overlooking the Lower Colorado River—the cliff of my earlier dreams. The property was available and I could afford it. I bought it, built a cabin on it, and moved into the woods within a year.

A big part of my move included setting aside the time and opportunity to find out who I am—the old-new me, the me that had been lost. Since the move, I've become quite clear as to who I am. I realize that part of my growth is attributable to the fact that I have a new sense of freedom in my life, and the introspective time that comes with that. My children are grown now, my work schedule is flexible, and I am at a wonderful age that allows me the wisdom of many winters while still having vitality and health. At sixty I feel wonderful, am exuberant, and only do what I want to do—well, mostly. It's a great time.

I've been learning that it's never too late to tap into your creativity unless you think it is. I don't think it's too late. So for me, it isn't. I am determined to create a life that reflects my desires. I choose to live a creative lifestyle as well as exercise any creative talents I have. So everything I do reflects my creative desires and wishes.

Looking back, I realize that everything I've done throughout my life has had a creative flair. No, I didn't become a professional artist, writer, or performer, but I always saw things from a different angle or added something that was unique. Maybe my creativity showed in the fact that I colored baked potatoes blue for a family picnic when I was a child. Or in the fact that I came to think of ADD in a new way, a positive way. Maybe most important of all has been the way in which I taught, and related to, children—as individuals.

My current creative activities cover the areas of music, art, dancing, community theater, performing arts, writing, animation, and music video. Of course, I don't do all of these activities at the same time. While I'm working on a few of them, the rest are lined up in my mind in a sequence of importance. I'm always mindful of opportunities to make progress when I meet someone with a skill I need or when a new idea comes to me.

I'm finding that the more I create, the happier I feel. The more involved I am with others, the more others speak of enjoying their creativity. We come together with our common interests and are fulfilled creatively.

I've come to believe that the benefits of creativity are even greater than I had previously realized. For example, when people are creating, they can't be fighting. I'm realizing that young people who are involved in creative pursuits don't have time to get into a lot of trouble. I also realize that people's outlooks on life are a whole lot better when they are using their creativity in some way.

One thing I can promise you is that you need to go ahead and create, even though you don't know whether or not you'll ever be able to sell your creations.

Write your short stories, poems, novels, or plays because they are inside you, craving to come out. Paint your pictures. Design your projects. Sing, dance, and make music. Play out your dramas on stage, film, and video.

Live a creative lifestyle and you will find a place for your creative interests on down the line. You will be the better for having created. And the world will be a better place because you will feel better and glow more brightly as a fulfilled creative person.

chaptertwo

What Is ADD?

N EW INFORMATION is surfacing daily about ADD. I find myself constantly revising the way I think about it and the way I talk about it. Although Attention Deficit Disorder is still its official name, I no longer call this type of brain wiring a disorder, or even a deficit. I'm not even comfortable calling ADD a difference. After all, people who do not have ADD aren't required by society to describe themselves as being "different"—even though they *are* different from those of us who are ADD.

So, as of the day I am writing this chapter, what I am willing and able to say about ADD is this: ADD is a neurobiochemical style of brain wiring.

This is just a statement of fact, not a judgment. It has no negative connotations.

It is not much different from my saying that I am a Caucasian female with blue eyes, an outgoing personality, and huge amounts of creativity. I am tall, have big feet, and am built more like an offensive lineman than a running back or receiver. I am very expressive but am also introspective and a dreamer. I come by all of these attributes via my genetic background. Both of my parents were probably ADD, and it's very likely that both of my sons are ADD, too.

These are simply statements, not judgments.

This particular style of brain wiring called ADD affects the ways in which people learn best, manage time, organize projects and materials, respond to their environment, communicate, need physical activity, relate to others, process information, and create. People with ADD do not do these things in a wrong way. They just do them in ways that are not always compatible with the surrounding culture. They do them in ways that are natural for them.

Traditionally, scientists and clinicians thought that people outgrew their ADD at puberty. Not so! You are born with it, grow up with it, and die with it.

Traditionally, only one girl for every seven boys was thought to have ADD. Now it appears that there is no difference in the incidence of ADD between males and females.

Traditionally, people were thought to *have* ADD. Now I believe people *are* ADD. That's just how we are wired. It affects how we see the world, how we do things, how we learn, and how we relate to other people. There are as many positive attributes to being ADD as there are negative, just as there are as many positive attributes to being non-ADD as there are negative.

But this is not to say that life is always as easy for people who are ADD as it is for those who are not. We live in a culture that is organized around non-ADD systems, and practices that favor non-ADD people. The educational system, business structures, cultural rules, laws, job expectations, and societal measures of success all favor a non-ADD style of being. In particular, the information age and the highly technical dehumanized nature of modern life have increased the discomfort level for many people who are ADD—people who are trying to live in a world full of details, paperwork, and numbers.

Once upon a time, before this age of electronic gadgetry, people learned their trades through apprenticeships, by watching and practicing the doing of their trade. And that is how people with ADD learn best, because they are kinesthetic learners. Today, lecturing, reading, and testing are the primary means of education. Due to this lack of hands-on experience, many people who are ADD do not fulfill their potential as students or employees.

Once upon a time when the seasons and the sun and moon served as people's watches, those who were ADD did quite well with "time management." They kept track of time by paying attention to how long it took to do a job. The content of what was being done determined how long people stayed on the job or in a conversation. Artificially segmenting time into minutes and hours is a different way of keeping track of time, and one that doesn't fit ADD people very well.

Both ways of marking time allow people to keep track of time and get things done, but the modern style of being chained to a date book and inflexible schedule does not favor people who are ADD. We are not less responsible or intelligent because we measure time differently than non-ADD people. We simply operate by a different clock than they do—and they operate differently than we do.

Unfortunately, people who are ADD are labeled as having time-management problems, while people who are non-ADD are not similarly labeled because they don't use nature to tell time.

Because we live in a world where most standards favor those who are non-ADD, we appear to be the ones who are different. We have been labeled disordered by those who are most like the cultural standards. Part of the problem stems from the fact that people with ADD usually don't care about labeling others, nor are we the ones who tend to write the diagnostic and statistical manuals.

If we did write the manuals and make the rules, ADD would never have been identified, and it would never have existed. Instead, we might have created CDD, Creativity Deficit Disorder; IDD, Intuition Deficit Disorder; or GSD, Goal Surplus Disorder.

How does that sound?

Diagnosing ADD

Because I am a realist, I know that those of us who are ADD need help to function effectively and live up to our potential in a culture that doesn't fit us. That's why a determination to see how you are wired is in order, so you can understand why you are experiencing difficulties and learn to make the necessary adjustments. But if you are "diagnosed" with ADD, do not believe that there is something *wrong* with you. Simply go through the process of diagnosis and then determine how you can best use your wonderful talents, gifts, and style to advantage in a very linear culture.

Few people as yet know how to determine whether people are ADD in a simple way. If you believe that you or a family member might be ADD, you need to find someone who has made it his or her business to learn about ADD and keeps up with the developments in the field. You need to find someone who has an open, nonjudgmental perspective on ADD and won't make you feel like there is something wrong with you—someone who values creative, innovative, and unusual ways of doing things.

Often the best diagnostician is someone who is ADD himself or has a child who is ADD. And that person is likely to be working in the field of mental-health or education, such as an educational diagnostician, counselor, psychotherapist, social worker, psychologist, or physician. Recently, teams of professionals have begun to come together to provide the well-rounded diagnostic services desired by people who are ADD.

An in-depth interview (about one to two hours) is usually adequate to determine whether or not you are ADD. Since ADD is present at birth and is genetically passed down through the family, the interview will cover your childhood as well as descriptions of relatives, including your parents and children. The diagnostician will ask about your experiences in school and the workplace, your interpersonal relationships, your behavior concerning everything from why you had certain accidents (was it from walking along the edge of the roof?) to your driving record. A brief physical history, including information about your use of addictive substances or tendency toward addictive behavior, is also important in determining whether or not you have an ADD brain-wiring style.

Testing really is not necessary. Some people prefer to use this method, though, and you may wish to be evaluated with psychological and educational tests. But if you are tested, be sure that an accurate history is also taken. Testing is a must, however, when there is evidence of an additional condition, such as a possible seizure disorder or other learning difference that the clinician wants to consider in making recommendations for medication and further intervention.

You may end up with a diagnosis of another condition as well as the determination that you are basically wired in an ADD way. ADD is not a diagnosis of exclusion. It can co-exist with conditions that are emotional and physical.

From your evaluation be sure to get not only a diagnosis but a written report that you can use to help you obtain reasonable accommodation in school and in your job. Finally, you need to be guided to what's next for you. You will want to find out what kinds of training will help you cope with the negative aspects of your ADD. How can you learn to better use your strengths? Is medication something that might help you and that you want to try?

Above all, stay in charge of yourself while working in partnership with a professional. Once you have discovered you are ADD, it will become clear how your creativity or potential for success may have been compromised. You'll find out how you can use ADD to your advantage, while factoring in the effects of ADD that you want to learn to control.

Let's suppose you were diagnosed as a child so you have known about your ADD for a long time. If you were fortunate you were provided with good guidance that helped you learn how to utilize your ADD positively and how to overcome any problems that it produced. If this is the case, by now you are probably well on your way to being a successful person, ADD and all.

If you were diagnosed as a child but were not helped to overcome your difficulties, or if you learned to feel badly about being ADD, you would do well to be rediagnosed now. New information and advances in working with ADD in addition to the guidance of people who are ADD will help you gain control of your life. You don't need to keep suffering because of ADD.

Once a determination of ADD is made, medication becomes an option. I've seen miracles with children and adults who suddenly can settle down, think one thought at a time, begin to act in ways that gain acceptance from those around them, and succeed in reaching goals. Unfortunately, I've also seen people who think medication for ADD means providing the "magic bullet" that will instantly cure every problem they've ever faced in life. They are in for a shock.

Medication provides a first step for many people diagnosed with ADD. But it is only one piece of a complex puzzle. Frequently, it buys time to learn management skills such as how to inhibit impulsivity, curb your temper, organize time and materials in ways that fit you, and find your own way of paying attention. Your job is to find your fit as an ADD-wired person in a culture that requires skills other than those that are natural for you. You will learn, given time, to adjust without losing your own identity. For some people, medication can help buy that time.

But under no conditions is medication to be used without training and education. I use the words *training* and *education* advisedly rather than *counseling*, which is not useful for ADD. Counseling is, of course, very helpful in dealing with the emotions and trauma that might result from your ADD issues. But to learn to manage the aspects of your ADD that cause you trouble, you will find training and education of greater benefit.

There are many kinds of help available to you. There are training programs that address specific ADD needs and books and workbooks that can help you learn to manage your ADD. And there are many, many support groups throughout the country to keep you updated on resources and provide camaraderie. On-line computer information is available if you are drawn to spend your time with your computer. You might also consider temporary coaching to assist you with the everyday steps and decisions you face. That kind of help can provide you with the opportunity to learn new ways of working and communicating, in order to get what you need out of life.

What ADD Is Not

I've been hearing and reading so much lately about ADD as an "excuse" that I want to start by saying, "ADD is not an excuse." It is a fact that ADD exists. Much of the way you see and react to the world depends on your ADD. That is just the way you are made.

It's kind of like being dealt a hand of cards. That's what you have to work with. ADD is an explanation—not an excuse. You get to use your assets as well as compensate for your vulnerabilities in the game of life. That's true whether or not you are ADD.

ADD does not mean you're crazy, inadequate, or in any way inferior to anyone else. You are only *different*, just as someone who is not ADD is *different* from you.

You are not stupid. In fact, people who are ADD are often much brighter than they are initially able to demonstrate in the formal educational environment. Your intelligence may show itself in ways other than making top grades in school.

The current tragedy in relation to ADD is that some educators and clinicians immediately label ADD and seek medication, creating a problem where one need not exist. Further misguided training to help the person become something he is not begins. That pulls the person farther off track. Trying to teach a fish to fly, rather than returning it to the water where it can learn to swim effectively is too often the solution sought by people who think *their* way of being is the way.

And all too often, the secondary problems associated with being ADD go unrecognized for what they are. If you are that fish who had been sent to flying school—the one who lost connection with your sense of self or opposed what was happening to you—you are in danger of developing behaviors that hurt you or that others think are a natural part of you. These include depression, oppositional/defiant behavior, anxiety, low self-esteem, and self-medicating behavior (such as substance abuse). These are common problems for people who are ADD, brought about by the frustration and anger that comes from being forced to fit into a system that just doesn't fit the needs or natural desires of someone who is ADD.

How sad! None of these reactions need happen. They are a result of mistreatment in an environment that doesn't fit. No more, no less.

Your job, though, is to believe in yourself and do two things. First, acknowledge, respect, and pursue your own innate interests and talents, taking responsibility for seeing that you share them with the world at large. This may mean making your living by those talents or it may mean enjoying them in addition to the work that provides you with the income you need to live a responsible life. (More on this in chapter 12.)

Your second obligation is to learn about the society you live in: the expectations, attitudes, beliefs, and rules. You don't need to agree with them. You don't need to respect all of them. But you do need to understand them and find ways to play the game.

Our culture is probably not going to meet you halfway, understanding your needs and reaching out to make things more equitable for you. You are the one who is going to have to reach beyond the midpoint in order to give others, who don't understand your talents and needs, what they think is appropriate. But you know the difference. Always be aware of the compromises you are making and why. That will save your neck and allow you to have a maximum amount of power in a situation that, though it doesn't fit for you, is the majority's way of doing things. Then you will gain in power yourself and can make your contribution to change cultural standards such as the educational system, legal system, or popular attitudes.

WHAT'S IN A NAME?

As I stated above, *ADD is not a disorder*. Historically, the people who researched, diagnosed, and created labels for people, putting them in little boxes on paper, were not ADD. That is simply not ADD behavior. Unfortunately, these labelers did not understand the meaning of what they were seeing or what they were doing. What they did understand was that children who did not do well in the current school system or in certain kinds of jobs could be diagnosed ADD.

What they didn't realize was that they were only looking at children in systems that didn't fit the way the children learn. Given a different style of education, such as apprenticeship and hands-on learning situations or job settings that incorporated flexibility and creativity, the same people actually did fine—even better than their non-ADD counterparts! But, nonetheless, they labeled the "misfits" as disordered.

It is time for this designation to change.

You are not disordered. In fact, you probably aren't deficient in many of the attributes normally associated with ADD, such as attention and organization. But you certainly do these things differently than non-ADD people—at times to your advantage and, true, at times to your disadvantage.

It wasn't very long ago that children diagnosed with ADD were thought to outgrow it at puberty. Then the literature began to reflect changing information about ADD in adulthood. At first, ten percent were thought to continue into adulthood with their ADD intact, then twenty percent. I recently saw an article stating that sixty percent of children with ADD continue to show symptoms into adulthood. But the reality is this: You are born with an ADD-style of brain wiring, you grow up with it, and you will have the privilege of dying with it. (While it is true that ADD symptoms can come about from head injuries, substance abuse, metal poisoning, or other outside causes, a condition called Acquired ADD, those are not the situations I am addressing in this book.)

I hope it won't be long until human differences are recognized and honored, rather than medicalized and disparaged. We can all contribute to this change by respecting ourselves as people who are ADD.

Each of us serves a wonderful role in the garden of life. All of our skills are necessary for the garden to bloom profusely. All we have to do is join forces to make a variegated arrangement that reflects the true beauty of life.

HOW THE ADD MIND WORKS

One of the most interesting aspects of the ADD mind has to do with how information is processed—how thinking takes place. There are two primary ways in which brains process information: the digital way and the analog way.

Digital refers to individual, discreet bundles of information. For example, if you have a digital clock, it reads one and only one time. On a digital clock it is either 9:27 A.M. or 9:28 A.M. You wouldn't look at a digital clock and say, It looks like it's about 9:27. It either is or it isn't. However, you cannot tell by looking at the clock whether it's just turned 9:27 or is almost ready to turn 9:28.

On an analog clock (the "old-fashioned" kind with the hour and minute hands), there's more clarity and more room for generalization. When the digital clock says 9:27, you might look at the analog clock and realize that it is midway between 9:27 and 9:28. On the other hand, you may choose to estimate the general time saying, it's nearly half past the hour of 9:00. There's more flexibility with the analog clock.

At one time digital and analog processing in the brain were related to the terms "left brain" and "right brain." However, that explanation has been considered overly simplistic. It indicated that each individual, or any type of activity, used either a digital or analog process. In reality, they both exist on a continuum of information-processing styles. While digital and analog processing might be at opposite ends of that spectrum, the middle contains infinite combinations.

As soon as you learn language, accept boundaries, and live within constraints, you do so primarily through the development of the symbolic and digital system. Current methods of socialization and education are responsible for programming the brain to function within a symbolic and structured world. This form of training better fits the person who processes information digitally.

Most people who are ADD tend to primarily be analog processors rather than digital processors of information. The culture in which we live not only favors people who are digital processors but *believes* that digital processing is superior to analog processing. Therefore, the way people who are ADD think and work is considered inferior. Thus the "diagnosis"—Attention Deficit Disorder.

The analog thinking process tends to be fluid, spatial, fluctuating, constantly changing with kaleidoscopic images and shifting forms. If your mind works this way, you are likely to notice backgrounds, moods, and new patterns rather than details. The feeling tones that surround even daily living are musical and poetic to analog processors. Emotions, visions, dreams, magic, novelty, and paradoxes provide the resources from which you draw to paint the experiences of your life. Analogies run rampant as a means with which to describe what you are trying to define or create. And the analog brain is tuned to survival in a natural environment. This translates into having "street smarts."

Analog thinking is present to a large degree in artistic expression, the ability to see the big picture and project expansively into the future. New leaps of imagination, the skill of sensing intricate feeling tones within your situation, along with subtlety of expression, are also a part of analog processing. The world is viewed in terms of a whole gestaltlike chunk, rather than in terms of details. Boundaries observed or created by digital thinkers are irrelevant or unimportant to analog thinkers, whose thrust of interest is in finding new and innovative ways of doing or seeing things or who see patterns that cross boundaries.

The digital processing system focuses on serial step-by-step sequences, rigid categories that differentiate detail, with considerable regulation to each single tick of the clock and each step taken. Digital thinking dominates speech, reasoning, sequential analysis, rational, logical, and abstract thinking.

Symbolic language that stands for something or codes information item-for-item is digital. No matter what type of clock you're using, time is measured in our culture in a digital manner rather than by moon cycles or seasons of the year. The accepted way to organize details and manage large projects tends to be reliant on the digital way of doing and maintaining things.

People, of course, do not fall neatly into one category or another, digital or analog. Some people will be evenly balanced between. Others, like myself, are almost exclusively analog processors and have very few natural digital skills. To be sure, I've learned some digital skills over the years. I had to in order to survive my education and in the work place. But none of it came naturally, and it was very, very hard for me to learn those skills. Keeping them up still requires my concentrated effort. When I'm tired, for example, the first thing that goes is any ability to organize systematically, including keeping track of time. But I can *always* see the big picture and create wonderful new castles in the sky, whether I'm tired or not.

RESULTS OF ANALOG VS. DIGITAL THINKING

I have a story I'd like to share with you. Shortly after I moved to Central Texas, a friend and I were standing on the edge of the cliff surrounded by the woods that has become my home. Looking skyward, we saw two hawks drifting on the air currents. Since we had met as volunteers who helped rehabilitate injured birds of prey, we shared an interest in identifying the hawks.

They were definitely not red-tailed hawks, so we stood gawking at the birds trying to figure out what they were. After a while my friend declared that she thought they were goshawks because of the window on the underside of each wing—a patch of white that stood out for her to see. No sooner had she said this than I started to laugh. I almost doubled over laughing.

What had I seen in my attempt to identify the hawks? I had been gazing, entranced, at the silhouette of their flight patterns against the blue sky. I'd had a wonderful experience that I could write a whole story about. I felt better for having viewed the hawks. I felt their "hawkness." In no way had I gained any information that would have been useful in helping to identify the hawk species. Yet my intent had been to identify them—not to have a creative, euphoric experience.

My friend is a registered nurse whose house is in order. She can find things most of the time, does beautiful patchwork quilts and has created a living habitat in her backyard with the proper balance of plants, water, and shade for the living creatures that inhabit it.

In contrast, I have a pretty, artistic home. To the outsider's eye it is definitely not in order. I paint and design one-of-a-kind craft pieces that I dream up on the spot. I find it beyond me to do any gardening because I can't keep track of what needs to be planted where, or pruned or watered when. Thank goodness the woods look great without my intervention. But then, that's why I live there.

My friend is predominantly a digital processor. I am overwhelmingly an analog processor. We share interests but go about managing and expressing our interests in very different ways.

Not only is it important to understand how your mind works, it's important to understand how friends' and coworkers' minds work if you are to do anything together. And each of us needs to develop an appreciation for the style of processing that is not our predominant mode. One is not better than the other. They are only different, designed to do different things.

Certainly living in a world that has as much complexity as our modern culture requires simple, straightforward ways to proceed and keep track of things. If you want or need to work efficiently, you need to progress in a digital or linear fashion. If your job requires you to sell more widgets than the competition, you may wish to find the quickest way to get from point A to point B. Or when you need to find one written document out of a whole library full of documents, you need a system that is direct and efficient.

When a linear (digital) mind is faced with a problem to solve, it begins to sift through the avalanche of information one point at a time considering the impact each piece of information might have on the problem. When one point is discovered, then the mind begins to scan in a similar manner for the second piece needed to fully solve the problem. Each point is lined up next to the others, until a solution is reached that fits the needs of the problem.

So, for example, suppose you lived near Austin, Texas, and needed to go to Dallas for a meeting and to pick up numerous boxes of books and bring them home to Austin in the shortest, most economical manner possible.

If you were a digital thinker, you might first consider what mode of transportation to take. Having decided that a plane is faster than a bus, train, or car, you would move on to the second point, which is to determine exactly what you need to take with you. You would then consider the weight of what you have to ship and probably discover that the cost of using air freight to send the boxes of books is too expensive for your budget. Or you might realize that the time it takes to drive to the airport, fly, rent a car, and proceed to the place of your meeting in Dallas takes almost as long as it would take you to drive the whole distance. Next, you would methodically look at all your options and then make a decision. And all of this would be done before you actually made the trip.

In contrast, the analog thinker is not likely to do this preplanning. The analog thinker might concentrate on how much he likes to fly or that he's accumulating frequent-flier miles. This might leave him with the impression that flying would be preferable. Research to determine the actual cost of shipping the books probably wouldn't be part of the decision. So, the analog thinker might book airline reservations on impulse, only to discover later that flying was not the best choice.

Somewhat embarrassingly, I discovered that a round trip from Austin to Dallas to Austin by air was only one hour shorter than driving. But I discovered that only after I had flown from Austin to Dallas. When I got to Dallas, I had no transportation and I had to pay to ship the books back to Austin, when I could have carried them as freight for free in the back of my pickup truck. Did I figure any of this out ahead of time? Of course not. It was only after several trips and the frustration of not having my own transportation in the city that it began to *feel* like driving was preferential to flying. I never did sit down to figure out what would be most efficient.

Fortunately, I usually prefer to drive because I can dream, look at the scenery, and relax. I no longer consider flying the relatively short distance. I realize there definitely is something to be said about digitally processing one's way through a problem. I just wish I would sometimes consider using it ahead of time!

On the other hand, if I have a creative story to write, I find that I'm very glad I am an analog thinker. As a member of a performing arts group in Austin, I received the assignment to create a descriptive poem about the various stages of life—and I needed it for the next day. I understood the type of poem I needed to write and simply tossed it in the back of my mind as I continued to do the other things that were on my schedule for the day.

That evening, as I sat on the edge of my cliff, I heard the first line of the poem, "Don't You Know!" I saw images in my mind of myself as a child and how I got off track from what I had loved then, such as watching the angels and fairies, climbing trees, and wearing boots and blue jeans. "Don't you know" kept playing through my mind as I recalled each precious situation that had made up my life and living experience. I saw how the heart's desires of my childhood had been quashed. Then I instantly saw how I had returned many years later to everything I once loved. In my reverie I realized that a hidden part of me had never lost my dreams and had worked to help me return to what is truly important to me. So the losses and the reunited dreams and desires each became a part of the magic of my life, Don't you know!

Then I simply wrote out the poem my mind had previewed for me.

The next day someone asked me, "How did you write your poem?" I answered, "It wrote itself."

Once the request for a certain type of poem is made to me, the poem within me that fits the agenda takes on a life of its own. I only have to write down what plays through my head. I do not consider this thinking—at least it's not linear thinking. Figuring out the most efficient route between Austin and Dallas gives me a headache, and I always forget key factors. But writing poetry this way never makes my head hurt. In fact, it makes me feel wonderful. And I rarely forget key ingredients to a creative writing assignment.

Yet I make a living in a world that requires me to deal with issues better solved by digital thinking processes. That makes life hard sometimes, because I really don't do that very well. On the other hand, I know several people who are the exact opposite of me, and I feel sorry for them. They have CDD, Creativity Deficit Disorder, and I'm sure their heads hurt if they have to create a story or speak extemporaneously.

Consider the situation of assessing whether or not a person is ADD. Professionals who are digital processors usually want to give tests and collect data piece by piece. Professionals who are analog processors prefer to hear the person's story and use their intuition to "diagnose" ADD, often simply knowing by feel whether or not a person is ADD.

Both professionals are likely to arrive at the same diagnosis, assuming they view ADD in the same way. But their methods will be quite different. Licensing boards and academic/research-oriented professionals sometimes don't realize the value and accuracy of both methods. These digital processors too often have IDD, Intuition Deficit Disorder, and so don't realize the power and accuracy of intuition.

Ironically, if I really put my mind to it, I can identify the specific cues that told me whether or not someone is ADD. But why struggle so hard to isolate those cues one at a time when I come to the same conclusion by viewing the person as a whole and using my intuition? I shouldn't need to prove, cue by cue, what I already know to be true. I know that analog processing works best for me and brings me the results I need.

For example, I recently had a training program that I wanted to sell. A friend of mine, who is a digital processor, suggested I do some marketing research at the nearest university to determine the value of my program and the best way to go about selling it.

At the sound of those words my stomach clutched into knots and my skin felt instantly clammy. I doubted that I could go through the movements of following those suggestions. But I also sensed I would not find out what I needed that way and would not end up any closer to my goal of selling the program.

Instead, I went about my daily business while keeping my goal in mind, selling my training program. Sure enough, it wasn't long before I bumped into three different people on three different days in three different settings, each of whom might be prospective buyers. As we shared information and goals, I assessed whether or not my training program fit their needs and whether or not their resources fit my needs.

After I made my determination in each case, I figured out a way to take the next step by involving them in working with the program. If any of these people feels comfortable with the program and enjoys using my material, I will probably have a potential deal. As to the details of the actual sale, I have every confidence that we'll work out a creative solution that will benefit both parties. Anything is possible when people's goals match, and the creative doors are opened to reach a solution in which everyone wins.

I've discovered that traditional research and business plans can often be a waste of time for analog thinkers. I've never gotten anywhere using those digital methods. To be sure my route often looks circuitous—but it works for me in the end.

My way is not for everyone, though. A linear person needs to take a linear route to solving problems. It makes no sense to say that he should just let things happen and watch for synchronistic circumstances to occur. That may not work for him. But he's not inadequate because of that. He's just different.

One of the problems for people who are ADD is our culture's very strong belief that digital problem solving is better than analog. From a very early age we are reinforced if we do things in a linear way, and we are told that there is a better way to do things if we are analog.

Consider Alex, the son of a friend of mine. Alex was about twenty months old when he sat down one day and organized his blocks into groups by color and size. His adult cousin, who had walked into the room at that time, gave him tremendous positive feedback saying, "What a great job you've done, Alex. How smart you are." She then told Alex's mom how smart and "advanced" he was.

That image—being praised for sorting things into small, homogenous groups—stayed with Alex, who is, of course, smart. But what if the cousin had come in and seen him mixing sugar and flour in a bowl, discovering how that mixture felt to his fingers. He might have figured out different ways to squish the mixture through his fingers or experimented to see how different the mixture looked when dropped onto the table from different heights.

In all likelihood, Alex the young scientist or sculptor would not have been labeled smart, nor would his mom have been complimented on her child's outstanding talents. His actions might even have been considered a behavior problem.

Categorizing things by details was just natural for Alex. For another child it would have been natural to experiment with the pattern that flour makes when it is poured on the floor. Both children would be smart, but their kinds of "smartness" differ. Generally speaking, our society is able to recognize one of these types of intelligence but not the other.

What kind of person are you? Do you wince when you think about the many times your experiments got you in trouble? Do you think of yourself as less smart than other people who can easily categorize, strategize, and research problems? Do you get defensive when linear people look down their noses at you even though you know you are as right about things as they are?

Ask yourself these questions and then take a stand to support the natural way you are. Believe in the value of *your* way and use it to accomplish what you want in the world. There's no need to put others down. Just recognize that differences are wonderful and equal.

Types of ADD

Those of us who are ADD do not make up one homogenous group, although we do share many common attributes. Over the years I've noticed three main types of ADD: Outwardly Expressed ADD, Inwardly Directed ADD, and Highly Structured ADD. Each of these three has strengths and weaknesses in terms of surviving and functioning effectively in the world as it is. Each displays commonly identified ADD traits in different ways. Identifying which form of ADD a person has makes it easier for me to figure out what that person needs—and why someone does what he does in the way that he does it.

Outwardly Expressed ADD

Candice is a super saleswoman. Artistically talented, she constantly comes up with new products and ideas. Her enthusiasm for anything new inspires her customers. And, usually, her ideas are good. For example, when she was designing a marketing campaign for a local politician, she completely turned his image around from a quiet egghead who was out of touch with his constituency, to a sensitive person who cared about the people he wanted to serve and had solid plans for helping them meet their needs. She got straight A's as an image shaper.

Later Candice started her own mobile pet-grooming business. Up until then, people in her area had to take their pets across town in inclement weather with children in tow or at inconvenient hours. When she couldn't manage to get her pet groomed at her convenience, she noticed a need for a mobile service. So Candice dropped other projects she was bored with, bought a van, had it redesigned inside and went into business. People loved her idea, and it definitely met a need in the community.

Unfortunately, however, Candice was out of business in a year because she couldn't manage the scheduling or keep track of her records. Her idea was great. But her management left a lot to be desired.

Over the years Candice has held many jobs, sometimes working in sales for a company and sometimes starting her own business. Although she prefers self-employment, she has often had to return to working for someone else because, when she was left on her own, her businesses tended to get off track as her paperwork and planning didn't get done.

She also had a problem with her temper. Coworkers knew not to cross Candice, who is really a cream puff at heart. But with little patience for office politics, Candice wasn't immune from telling off the boss, or anyone else for that matter. Now in her early forties, Candice has her temper fairly well under control—at work at least. She figures she's lost out too many times because of impatience and impulsivity and is trying very hard to keep her mouth in check.

Candice is typical of one type of person who is ADD. Very creative, outgoing and overachieving, she is spontaneous and able to "go in for the kill" with impeccable timing when a deal needs to be closed. But that same high level of sensitivity and intuition that lets her quickly and accurately assess business situations also causes her to suffer hurt when she is around a painful situation or person who is critical, blunt, or abusive.

Candice has Outwardly Expressed ADD. I call people with that type of ADD the Active Entertainer. Many successful people in show business, public relations, sales, and any high-risk business are wired in this way. Anyone can see everything they are doing or thinking or feeling. It's all out there for the world to view. Good of heart, this type of person leaves little to the imagination. However, quick reactions also mean a tendency to job hop and not stay in relationships for very long. Living in terror of getting bored, people with Outwardly Expressed ADD are often seen stirring things up.

When someone with this type of ADD utilizes her innate talents and gifts, she is likely to be highly successful in life. If you are wired this way, you may already be using your ADD to advantage. If, however, you haven't yet discovered your identity and your innate talents and gifts, it is likely that you have gotten into a fair amount of trouble—possibly including getting fired or even ending up in jail—for acting impulsively and being disruptive, especially if drugs or alcohol are involved. No one will doubt your level of frustration, but neither will society feel sorry enough for you to tolerate your inadequacies.

If you are a person with Outwardly Expressed ADD, you might be more concerned with getting a job done than with spending the time it takes to do a quality job. When you are confronted with your own slap-dash job, you may be inclined to blame the other guy rather than reassessing what you might have done better.

People with Outwardly Expressed ADD tend to be extremely active, both physically and verbally. They feel severely confined when asked to stay seated, sit still or walk at a leisurely pace. If you have this type of ADD, you are probably very familiar with the feeling of wanting to get on with the show and not stay in one place too long. If you can channel your activity level properly, you can really accomplish a lot. If not, your activity level can get you into a lot of trouble. You'll have to decide for yourself which way to go on this one.

If you have Outwardly Expressed ADD, your emotions ride the waves from crest to trough depending upon what is happening in your life at a given moment. With lots of childlike innocence you may reign eternally hopeful even in the presence of a sinking ship. Then when, to your surprise, the ship sinks, you are devastated, not having seen it coming.

I understand what you are going through because I have a lot of this type of ADD to contend with. I love it—but it does cause me trouble at times.

Inwardly Directed ADD

Matthew tinkers. He builds all kinds of things—inventions for easier living, fountains and houses for birds and people—and he dreams. Since he was a little boy, Matthew could be seen staring off into space. When asked what he was doing, he'd reply, "Thinking." Then the next day he'd arrive with something that he'd drawn or made. One time it was a small broom made out of pine boughs that he'd constructed to sweep a friend's fireplace. Another time he sketched a design for a go-cart that eventually won a prize in a school contest.

Though he didn't always finish his schoolwork, Matthew did manage to complete high school. He chose not to go to college, however, although he certainly had the intelligence for it. He felt "formal" education got in the way of his learning. He knew what he wanted to learn, and he knew how to find any information he needed.

Matthew could look at a building project or problem and immediately see the whole picture. He would then begin to play with ideas for solving the problem. He called it "puttering around" in his mind. Sometimes he would then tinker with various ways to produce a prototype to solve a problem. People who didn't understand how Matthew's mind worked would try to get him to make a plan or an outline. When he was young, that frustrated him. Now he knows that's just a waste of time for him.

For a long time, though, Matthew's frustration fed his feelings of inadequacy. He became quite depressed as a young adult and felt like a failure as he watched his classmates take off in their careers. He even blamed himself for not trying harder.

Depressed, trying many different ways to make a living by doing whatever came along, Matthew had little time for any social life. Although he didn't mind that a lot because he was fairly shy, he did like company. He had one friend, though, who liked to "mess around" with wood, repairing used furniture and building anything he thought he could sell.

The two spent many evenings together, not saying much but enjoying keeping each other company while working on their individual projects. Matthew told his friend about his ideas for building homes using wood and stone. He figured he might never have an opportunity to do the building he wanted to do, but his dream wouldn't go away.

Then one day, the father of his "messing around" friend asked him if he would please take charge of building a house—one the man had in his mind. He hadn't been able to find anyone who could capture his dream. But after listening to his son talk, he had a hunch that Matthew might be the very person he was looking for.

Matthew not only captured this man's dream in wood and stone but did it in an economical and timely manner. Finally, Matthew began to realize that he wasn't so inadequate after all. He was on his way to a career that fit him.

The main hitch that Matthew ran into was keeping track of his business—the records, pieces of paper, and money. He also became restless from time to time if the house he was building didn't tax his creative talents. Boredom, which came from doing something he already knew how to do, conflicted with his desire to make a substantial living. This became even more stressful after he met a woman he thought he could settle down with. He vacillated between taking on the responsibility of being a married man and being free to accept only those jobs that he really wanted to do.

When Matthew couldn't make up his mind about getting married, his girlfriend became anxious and began to nag him. Soon their relationship soured, but Matthew seemed unable to let go of it. Finally she handed him an ultimatum which he didn't answer. She left, taking his silence for a "no."

Matthew has Inwardly Directed ADD. He is what I call a Restless Dreamer.

Many people who are artists, artisans, craftsmen, and inventors are wired with this form of ADD. The old-fashioned engineer who can jury-rig anything, the mechanics, builders, and technical people of the world, often fit into this category. Many people who enjoy working outdoors, or with plants and animals, have Inwardly Directed ADD. Finally, many people drawn to service-oriented jobs that make use of empathy and sensitivity, including teachers and counselors, are using the talents that came with their Inwardly Directed ADD.

It's often hard to tell what someone with Inwardly Directed ADD is thinking because talking may not be their forte. But you often find this type of person communicating through their work. A glance will acknowledge that what one person is doing is appreciated by another. Subtle social cues are often missed by their less sensitive coworkers. But don't ever underestimate the quiet dreamer who sees a whole lot more than is communicated openly.

If you are wired in this way, your biggest problem may be depression. "Stuffing" your feelings, rather than getting them out, won't give you a chance to express anger, frustration, and helplessness. You need to realize that glitz and dog-and-pony-shows aren't the only ways to success. It could be that your quieter way is just fine. But you do need to stand up for yourself and your way of doing things. Just as Matthew finally learned that his way was okay, you, too, must come to believe in yourself—even in the face of another's rejection.

You are likely to stay too long in any given situation, job or personal, whereas your counterpart with Outwardly Expressed ADD tends to not stay long enough. Indecision, procrastination, and "dreaming around" can block you from moving toward implementing your dreams. A lot of these reactions, however, result from your not believing in yourself—your talents, unique ways of doing things, and your dreams.

Though you are not hyperactive physically, and certainly not hyperverbal, you probably hate being tied to a desk. Restless is a good word to describe what you feel. You may rarely be still. But even your movement is probably subtle as you shift weight and walk around quietly.

Ultimately, pessimism can get you down, so you will need to make a real effort to look on the bright side of things. With the dreams you hold inside, all you need to add is belief in yourself, and you can become the winner you were always meant to be. Don't stop dreaming. Teaming up with someone who can sell your dreams may be just the solution you've been looking for. Keep your eyes open!

Highly Structured ADD

Gwen has her own company. She has found her fit in the age of computer technology. She organizes everything in her life by using her computer, so much so that a scrap of paper rarely crosses her desk. E-mail has replaced letters and even faxes. Computer bulletin boards often bring her together with the people she needs to spend time with in business and allow her to get answers at a moment's notice. The Internet has become her main marketing tool.

Throughout school Gwen was the perfect student. She didn't mind doing homework, as long as the assignment was clear. The only time she really had trouble was when her science teacher told her to brainstorm for a week and then develop a science project, any project she liked. Gwen didn't have any idea where to start her thinking, and she panicked. She told her teacher that the assignment was stupid and that it needed to be redefined.

The teacher took mercy on Gwen and gave her two projects to choose from, along with a set of guidelines for proceeding. Within this structure—with a small, fixed number of variables—Gwen was able to be comfortable and creative.

As an adult Gwen's hobbies include quilting and folk painting, both of which are highly structured activities. Her house is orderly and she becomes upset when company comes and leaves a path of chaos behind. It takes her a long time to get things back in order. She doesn't understand why people can't do one thing at a time and put things back where they got them when finished.

Gwen is not an unkind person. She just hates disorder. It makes her feel bad, even frightens her because she doesn't have a clear picture in her mind of how to regain control of the situation and restore order. She has a hard time creating a structure for herself.

Her friends call her a perfectionist, and she supposes she is. She wishes everyone would be that way. Life would be a lot simpler then. This need almost cost her a marriage when she tried to apply her values and principles to her husband, a fairly laid-back person. And it's a good thing he was relaxed, or he probably would have left the marriage. He did almost walk out when Gwen's need for control took a scolding form. He didn't mind if she wanted things highly organized, but he *did* mind when she started to take over his life and talk down to him.

Gwen discovered that they each had to have areas in which to take responsibility and have supreme control. That way, they could each handle their own affairs the way they wanted to in their specific area and leave the other person alone. Gwen, who loved her husband and didn't want to lose him, realized she had to go along with this plan.

Gwen has Highly Structured ADD. She is the kind of person I call a Conscientious Controller. Many people in the military, who do accounting and financial planning, or who pilot aircraft or perform intricate, delicate procedures fall into this category. Any job requiring extreme attention to detail and precision serves as a comfort for the Conscientious Controller.

If you have Highly Structured ADD, you typically appear to be very controlling. But that's not because you're a bad person. Rather your problem lies in not being able to create a structure easily. Once a structure is in place, you need to hold tight to it, which includes expecting others around you to do the same.

As one man I knew explained it, "No sooner do I get everything in place than someone or something changes one aspect of it, and everything is destroyed. There I sit in a pile of rubble so that I have to rebuild the whole thing all over again, piece by piece. And that takes a very long time, a lot of strenuous energy, and a lot of worrying that I won't get it right.

Often feeling overwhelmed, people with Highly Structured ADD are likely to be fairly rigid in their thinking, have quick tempers and worry obsessively. As the person with Highly Structured ADD tries to regain control, he tends to find fault with others. His mind is telling him, "If only I can lay the blame on someone else, then I might have a chance to regain my equilibrium."

This type of person obviously has trouble cooperating with others. Negotiation is not easy for him. And, I promise you, with this type of person around, there can only be one boss.

The more unstructured the coworker, the more anxious, frustrated, and judgmental the person with Highly Structured ADD becomes. Brainstorming, freewheeling creativity, and trial-and-error ventures make this person nuts. Even in his creative ventures, the creativity will follow a definite, controlled plan or proven formula.

Communication is a problem for this type of person because he has trouble listening. He is so fearful of not being heard that he tends to say the same thing over and over again, and his excessive talking *at* another person leaves no room to determine the effect of what is being said. Some of this repetition is related to the biochemistry of the person's brain. It is difficult for this type of person to change gears from one activity to another—including changing from speaker to listener. Being a listener also requires constant adjustment to what the next response will be. That's hard if you're Highly Structured ADD.

If, however, you want a job done to perfection, the over-organization of the Conscientious Controller may just be an asset. Certainly in life-threatening situations or whenever a great deal is at stake, over-organization, control, and hyperfocusing are an asset. If you are able to sit at a computer screen intently focusing on a program, you may just be the first one to solve a difficult problem. And you can always sleep the next day.

Hypoactivity, also an attribute of ADD, is most likely to show up in this type of person. Thus a steady hand may repair watches, stay within the lines demanded of stylized painting, or keep the straight lines and tiny stitches necessary for intricate quilting.

Combined Forms of ADD

The faces of ADD do indeed look different on the surface from one form of ADD to the next. But underneath, each person has some type of compromise to the same brain center. Just as a frenetic weasel anxiously scurries about, a cat may sit transfixed, watching the opening of a mouse hole for the appearance of the prize he seeks. You won't be fooled by external appearances if you realize that underneath the surface lies a maze of complicated, yet, in some ways, incredibly simple, brain neurochemistry that dictates the appearance of assets and liabilities.

You may see aspects of yourself in one, two, or all three forms of ADD. Any combination is possible.

For example, Monte has a combination of Highly Structured and Outwardly Expressed ADD. An emergency-room physician, he studied obsessively at medical school, and took top honors. As long as he knows what is expected of him, he's in fine form. The tight structure of the medical school curriculum made him feel confident.

When Monte first left the confines of schoolwork, though, he felt insecure until he learned procedures he could count on time after time after time. He made copious notes and preferred situations in which clear-cut guidelines were present for him to follow.

Because he also has an outgoing, high-risk-taking aspect to him, he found he was especially attracted to emergency room medicine. He loved the excitement, and his flamboyance made him a good leader of a team where the sequence of lifesaving duties was clear cut. His thinking became extremely clear in these situations, and he was able to work nonstop until the patient was out of danger.

Monte knew himself well enough to know that he could never go into anesthesiology or dermatology, which would confine him, trapping his hyperactive body. He also knew that he needed the absolute line of control offered by a triage team where he could be in charge. A perfectionist, he used his ADD profitably.

As you can see, each category of ADD, and every possible combination of those forms, has assets and liabilities. The bottom line is that you need to find out how your ADD manifests itself so you can find your fit—so you can discover your strengths and talents and determine how to best use them. When you've accomplished that, you've set yourself up to be a winner.

ADD is as good as it is bad, as easy as it is difficult. Just as a non-ADD person must face liabilities because he is non-ADD, you can compensate for your down sides and make good use of your strengths. Teaming with others who are different from you, as you mutually respect one another's abilities, will make a whole that can make a difference for everyone involved.

chapter three

Your Natural Creativity

L OOKING DOWN my street one Sunday, I noticed the activities of three of my neighbors. The middle-aged man who lives a couple of houses away sat on his porch swing staring into space. Every now and again he nodded his head or made a few notes on a piece of paper that he'd pulled out of his pocket.

The young woman next door was making dolls. She designs and constructs specialty dolls that she sells at Renaissance fairs and holiday markets. I often see her picking up sticks and flowers as she walks in the woods near my home. She weaves these into the costumes of her dolls, making each unique.

A dozen kids surrounded my third neighbor. I noticed that they were doing calisthenics and then running in relays. Then I saw them huddled together, talking excitedly as they flailed their arms around. Finally, my neighbor jumped up with the kids following suit. They made swooping movements and took standing and sitting positions like statues. When he called, "Freeze," they did. He moved between them, changing the direction of an arm or the way it was bent. Everyone seemed to be having a wonderful time.

Now I ask you, which of these neighbors is being creative?

My reply is, "All of them."

It's pretty easy to recognize that the doll maker is creative. But she is not the only one. My porch-swing neighbor, who seems to be day-dreaming, is a mechanical engineer in the process of working out a creative design for a manufacturing process. He mentally works out the prototypes in his mind, gets new ideas to solve the problems presented to him at work, and generally spends most of his time as a creative designer.

My third neighbor is training junior-high kids to perform in half-time programs. He is mixing dance with athletic training and cheerleading. He has never had any special training in any of this but discovered that he loved working with young people. He also realized that most of these kids didn't have much to do and were starting to get into minor trouble because they were bored. He also realized that the junior varsity sporting events didn't have any entertainment at half-times.

So, aware of two sets of needs that might intersect, he put the word out that he was going to hang out on Sunday afternoons in an attempt to do something about the boring state of affairs. After everyone spent time complaining, he guided the discussion around to what they could do about it. He suggested they just try some things. He noticed what the kids seemed to have the most fun doing and developed half-time routines from that. Then he introduced creative practice sessions, which often ended up with a lot of fun and laughter.

The students realized they needed a lot of energy and muscle if they were going to look good, so my neighbor helped them find a way to work out that wasn't too boring and didn't cost money. Together they all began to choreograph some routines, though they never completely gave up their free-form fun as one part of the entertainment.

Each of these neighbors is a highly creative individual, though only the doll maker thinks of herself that way. The mechanical engineer occasionally realizes he is an innovative designer, but he doesn't use the term "creative" to describe himself or what he does. And, to be sure, the "coach" would probably laugh if I suggested that he is a creative person. He sees himself as someone who helps kids.

There are so many faces of creativity. In this chapter I hope to broaden your perception of what creativity is and how it is reflected—in yourself as well as in other people. In the end you'll discover everyone is creative, including you.

THE DEVELOPMENT OF CREATIVITY

When I contemplate the fact that everyone is creative, I find myself thinking about ourselves as babies. From the moment a child is born, the very process of living demands creativity—the way in which we express our uniqueness and the way in which each of us adapts to the surroundings in which we find ourselves.

No two of us are exactly alike. Even identical twins quickly demonstrate differences that parents can identify.

Creativity is not learned. It comes automatically. Its roots emanate from deep within us, shaped by our physical, emotional, mental, and cognitive differences. Creativity is a complex mix of all these factors.

As babies and young children, our differences can be affected positively or negatively by our parents and other adults. For creativity to continue to show itself and to grow, it needs freedom. But even if your creativity ran up against blocks and barriers, I promise you, it is still in you. It really never goes away.

Creativity involves certain characteristics that are familiar to all of us, characteristics that we each have to some degree. For example, you may have a lot of originality but not much independence. The next person may be attracted to complexity and its mysteries, be very intuitive, curious, and enjoy ambiguity but not particularly like to take risks. A third person may not worry about rules, be inventive, enjoy brainstorming and have a lot of psychic ability, but not be able to separate things and recombine them into new wholes.

Each of these characteristics is a part of how I define creativity. You might want to check yourself against this list and see which ones you have.

_____ ORIGINALITY

_____ INDEPENDENCE OF THOUGHT

_____ INDEPENDENCE OF ACTION

_____ ATTRACTION TO COMPLEXITY AND ITS MYSTERIES

_____ INTUITION

_____ TAKE RISKS

_____ CURIOSITY (MENTAL OR PHYSICAL)

_____ FLEXIBILITY

_____ ENJOYMENT OF AMBIGUITY

_____ NO WORRY OR CARE ABOUT RULES

_____ ENJOYMENT OF BRAINSTORMING

_____ PSYCHIC ABILITY

_____ ABILITY TO TAKE SEPARATE THINGS AND COMBINE THEM IN NEW WAYS

How did you come out? I wonder whether you've previously thought about yourself as creative. Since many of these characteristics are typical of creative activity, if even one of these characteristics applies to you, that means you have at least one attribute of creativity. And I bet you have more than that. There are probably many aspects of your personality that are related to long-forgotten areas of creativity in you.

When and How Does Creativity Develop?

From birth to eighteen months, you (like every other child) had one major emotional task—to develop a sense of trust that your needs would get met. Trust is the first of five components of the Core Components of Human Nature, and it is critical in order to be able to feel secure when you are vulnerable.

As a baby and toddler, you soon learned whether or not you could count on the adults around you to meet your needs and protect you from harm. From then on, and to this very day, your ability to open your heart to other people and new situations is dependent on how well you weathered those crucial early months.

Your sense of trust served as a foundation from which creativity could show itself. If you were not raised in a trusting environment, one in which you received enough consistent care that was supportive rather than abusive or neglectful, you began to close off emotionally as a very young person. As a result, your creativity will have a hard time showing itself. Trust serves as a foundation that makes it safe for you to remain open and expressive—key attributes of creativity.

From eighteen months to three years, your emotional focus shifted from building a sense of trust to beginning the physical and emotional separation from your caregivers—so you could start to uncover your identity as an independent person. By taking your first telltale steps away from Mom or Dad, you risked going out on your own. Neither getting too far away nor being held back, you learned a new kind of safety-independence. As you did, you noticed yourself, perhaps for the first time, and that self reflected your individuality and uniqueness.

The way in which you were raised during this stage was critical to your development of an identity that fits you. If you were raised by parents or caregivers who believed in the "empty vessel" philosophy, you were considered a vessel into which acceptable behaviors, attitudes, and expectations were stuffed. (Often, this process is called socialization.) For example, if you are a woman, you may have been expected to sit still and wear dresses as a little girl and have your hair fussed over—irrespective of the fact that you might have preferred to climb trees in jeans and have short hair that was easy to fix and didn't get tangled in those trees.

If the behaviors, attitudes, and expectations stuffed into your "empty vessel" fit you, then you would have emerged from this method of child rearing without a lot of scars and with an identity that fairly well approximated your innate identity. If not, you are likely to have doubts about yourself, not really knowing who you are or what you like.

The other way to raise children is by the "gardening" approach. If you were raised this way, someone took a close look at you to see how you were made. You were given nurturing and support and put in environments that fit you. So if you liked to climb trees, you were dressed appropriately and given the opportunity to do so. If you preferred to stay in the shade and read a book, that was okay, too. If you occasionally misbehaved, you were shown the right way to behave, but you were never brutalized or shamed. A gardener does not chop down the whole shrub when it sends out a sucker. Only the sucker is removed. Watered, cultivated, and given a trellis to grow on, your garden grows beautifully. People are no different.

If you were raised with the empty-vessel approach, then all the beliefs, behaviors, and attitudes that were stuffed inside you probably trapped your natural creativity. On the other hand, if you were raised with the gardening approach, your natural creativity would have emerged well and healthy and would have shown itself early.

Parents of children raised with the gardening approach usually see their child's natural creativity for the first time before the age of three. How exciting if that happened to you. You would have had an opportunity to show your interests, some of which you may still have to this day.

Turning three meant that you moved into a new stage of development, one in which the core component that naturally demanded attention was a sense of competence. As a three-year-old, you were primarily interested in what you could do. You would have had a natural feeling that you could do anything. You would have been interested in the process of doing things, not the end result.

What is so wonderful about this stage is the fact that children naturally and normally have a feeling of being a competent person, that is, unless they were abused or neglected earlier. As a competent-feeling child you would have naturally wanted to experiment and express and expand your natural creativity. As a child with an ADD style of brain wiring, you are likely to have been a busy little person.

In the process of playing, you would have tried all kinds of things with no fear of failure or making mistakes, unless your experience had taught you to be afraid. Creativity at this stage is still about the process of doing things. What the finished creative product looks like is irrelevant to a three-year-old. If it remained irrelevant to those around you, you weren't criticized or didn't have your creativity put down.

Almost magically, you are likely to have gone through a transformation around the time you turned four. If you had a foundation of trust that your needs would be met by surrounding adults, a beginning sense of your identity, and a feeling of being competent, then at four, you would be ready to see just how much you could do for yourself. This is the emotional power-building stage—a stage that is a natural component of becoming a responsible person who gains appropriate control of your life without hurting anyone else.

This sense of emotional power means that you extended your control in relation to getting your *own* needs met, rather than being dependent on someone else to meet those needs. Rather than asking for help from a grown-up, you might have pulled the chair over to the counter, climbed up on it yourself, unlatched the cupboard door and gotten your own crackers down from the top shelf.

Your ability to develop a healthy, constructive sense of power depended on your learning the limits within which you could appropriately exercise your power. A fire is a wonderful thing when it is contained within a fire pit or furnace, it is destructive when it rages out of control. So, too, emotional power to get your needs met is wonderful as long as it is contained within generally accepted limits of civilization. That way, you get what you need, but not at another's expense.

In order to focus your creativity and make use of it, you need a well-developed sense of emotional power. When you were four and five years old, you were ready for your creative endeavors to become a little more goal-oriented. It's not that you would lose touch with the process of creation but that you would use that creation for some purpose.

One of the main reasons that adults don't know what to do with their creativity is that they did not develop a sufficient sense of emotional power as a child. When you stop to think about it, our culture as a whole has never made it through this developmental stage. Institutions and people in control frequently use power to control others rather than to get their own needs met without curtailing another person's right to do the same.

Education does not teach children to be in charge of what is best for them. Instead, educational goals are set and directed by the grown-ups. Because those goals often don't fit people who are ADD, you may have been made to do things many times that weren't particularly constructive for you—or were downright bad for you.

All of this impacted your learning how to manage both your own needs and your creativity, since you must be in a power position to release your own creativity. Remember that being creative opens you to your vulnerability. Your emotional power will help you protect yourself, to balance out that vulnerability. So you see how important it is to have a well-developed sense of power if you want to bring your creativity out into the open and make use of it.

From five to six, you went about the business of developing self-control. This was the stage when you took the values into yourself that you saw displayed by the important people around you. Having developed empathy for the first time, you truly wanted to do what you felt was *right* because you didn't want to hurt someone you cared about.

Ultimately, living with a value system that originates from inside yourself—so that you do things because you *want* to rather than because you *should*—will lead you to expressing your own true creative nature. That's because that true creative nature reflects truth within yourself. On the other hand, creativity will be blocked by trying to do something that does not originate from within yourself as a true desire.

"Shoulds" do not reflect authenticity for you as an individual. "Wants" do. You will automatically be more creative when you live from your own truth than when you mimic what others feel is right for you.

During that critical five- to six-year-old period, your perceptions also changed. Remember that at age three, you didn't care at all what your creative productions looked like because you didn't perceive your work in relation to models or standards. As a five-year-old, you suddenly were able to compare your work with those models and standards. At age five, you became able to see how your work compared with reality. But because your skills were fairly undeveloped, you could not yet approximate in your creations what you saw with your eyes. So when you went to draw a tree, your tree didn't look like your model. It bothered you at age five. You probably became discouraged even if no one said a negative word or did anything to stunt your creativity.

The whole trick at this stage was for grown-ups to reassure you that you would become more skillful so that in time you would be able to draw the tree the way you wanted to draw the tree. Unless someone reassured you, you may have found it hard to keep your creative expression alive and well. You were likely to have become very cautious and concerned about "getting it right." Inner judgments at this age probably arose to inhibit your creative expression. You needed lots of continued reassurance to keep your creative expression alive. If all went well you were given creative tasks that did not require a lot of skill or that didn't require you to match a standard. At best you were encouraged and given the hope that you would eventually be able to do what you wanted to do.

Finally, groundwork could have been effectively laid at this period that made whatever you did okay—a sort of no-holds-barred approach that encouraged an attitude that anything goes. You could learn that one thing is as good as another.

As you can see, each of these Core Components of Human Nature had a major effect on the health and well-being of your creativity. But what you need to know now is this: Regardless of how you got through these five initial stages, you can help yourself *now* to get what you didn't get earlier.

It is not too late to make up for any deficiencies. If you need to be more protective of your creations, you need to build your emotional power. If you didn't

42

have the opportunity to feel good about your competence, you can begin to experiment now. Every one of the core components is fixable. That is great news!

THE FUNCTIONS OF CREATIVITY IN CHILDHOOD

Creativity is a special gift that is natural and present in all of us as children. We were able to turn to our creative side to receive inspiration for growth and hope. We needed the alive, wonderful energy within us that could help us deal with a world that seemed foreign and often hurtful as we tried to learn how to fit into others' expectations.

I'm reminded of a woman I know who wasn't very happy with her family life as a child. She used to carry around a pink plastic notebook in which she wrote stories about families she invented. Everyone was happy almost all the time in these families she created. And when there was a conflict, the family was able to resolve it peacefully.

This woman's creativity expressed itself in childhood through writing—writing that was used to help fill something missing in her life. It gave her hope and inspiration. Oh, by the way, she grew up to be a writer.

I have come to believe that one of the main functions of creativity throughout our lives is to bring us in touch with a wonderful, supportive, invigorating, hopeful part of ourselves. It touches our dreams, encasing them so that we can feel them and use them to create a better world for ourselves.

I believe that our creativity is a reflection of our connection with a Higher Power—however each of us conceptualizes that power—and that our creative work flows from that highest, most truthful part of ourselves. Our creativity is like breath. It is life-giving and sustaining.

Creativity is a process that allows for transformation into anything we want to become. Our creativity is as unlimited as that Higher Power, ever re-creating itself. How wonderful to tap into that self-propelling aspect of Divinity. Each of us can truly create, in conjunction with our own conception of God, a life that reflects the aspects of ourselves that we wish to emulate. By envisioning who we are, how we see ourselves and what we want, we can create the very life that we desire.

The more you learn to believe in and release the creative aspects of yourself, the more you will affect your environment, creating one that is wonderful. And the more you release creatively, the more you will find within yourself the enormous amounts of talent and energy you possess. Try it. You may be as surprised as I have been.

Creativity also reflects our ability to play as a child, to lightly jostle the many elements that allow us to redesign the world around us. To play with an idea means to open our minds to create something new. To play in the world means we have given ourselves permission to go beyond stringent barriers that entrap us—such as the prison of doing things "just right."

Creative play allows us, in a sense, to create power in our lives. Creativity and play function very similarly. They allow the child you were and, later, the grown-up you became to change something. You may not have planned it that way, but on some level within you, you had a desire for change. You set that desire free in order to allow the change to occur.

Your creativity gave you a sense of power as a child. This happened within yourself in part through fantasy. But the effects were seen in your "real life" environment, too. It allowed you to have an effect on things around you. Others were affected by the new ways in which you interacted with them or your environment.

For example, consider the little girl who carried her notebook around, creating stories about happy families. Because she kept busy, she probably made fewer demands on her already stressed parents, which could have helped diffuse a difficult situation for all of them. Perhaps her siblings, too, were calmed by the direction that her creativity took her.

Remember Mr. Potato Head—the child's game that comes with a potato-shaped plastic head into which children can put a variety of noses, ears, mouths, and so forth? It's a kind of "design-your-own-head" game. Just as you can change Mr. Potato Head's face by inserting different plastic facial features, you can design a life for yourself by inserting different activities into your daily life.

THE CONNECTION: FROM CHILD TO ADULT

All of us carry our childhood experiences into adulthood.

All the experiences that you had during your early years are stored in your memory banks. Some experiences you remember vividly, while others are buried deep within you. But even the buried ones influence what you do now and how you feel.

If you had positive creative experiences as a child, you are likely to feel comfortable now with your creativity. If, however, you were forced for one reason or another to stuff your creativity down inside you and hide it from the world, you are likely to either feel uncomfortable now in situations that draw upon your creativity or to feel that you are not creative at all. Either way, you are being cheated.

Take Jason, for example. As a child he loved to tinker with stuff. Even as a preschooler, he took things apart around the house—the toaster, the garden gate, his grandpa's airplane models. As Jason grew up, he began to put things together. He was able to fix fences, broken furniture and machines, and generally repair almost everything. He especially liked to improvise when he made repairs, sometimes redesigning and improving the way the object was made.

Jason's parents and grandparents encouraged him. Once, when he redesigned the pump handle on the family farm, his grandfather bragged about it to his friends and invited his grandson to join them for breakfast at the local cafe. At this breakfast the local doctor mentioned that he was having trouble figuring out how to help one particular young patient. This bright boy was confined to a wheelchair and needed special mechanical help to communicate his thoughts. Jason, fifteen at that time, asked to take a look at the situation. He figured out how to rig a temporary solution until the doctor could find a more sophisticated method.

This experience so inspired Jason that he began to talk further with the doctor about other medical problems. He eventually decided to go to medical school. Jason specialized in the design and development of prosthetic and mechanical health care devices, and he became a highly successful professional in the physical medicine department of a medical school. Thanks to the support and encouragement he received as a child and a teen, Jason continued to use his inherent creativity to the advantage of many people. And he always loved his work.

Twila, on the other hand was not so lucky. As a young child she loved to dance and sing. Even before she could write, she directed the other preschool children in "dramas." She made up the plays, picked costumes for her actors and found other children to serve as an audience for her productions. As soon as she learned to write, she wrote dialogue for her actors and staged plays for the whole neighborhood.

Seeing her interest, her parents eagerly fawned over the talent demonstrated by their daughter. As soon as she was old enough, they signed her up for dancing and acting lessons. Then they started her with a piano teacher and a voice teacher. Soon Twila was busy every day and had little time for the love of her heart, putting on productions.

What had started out as play for Twila turned into work. And she was working all the time. Even school took a back seat to her lessons. Though very bright, she began to struggle in fourth grade when the expectations on her increased. She was getting tired of all the responsibilities that she was carrying and began to cut back in the one area that her parents were not paying attention to—school.

Worst of all, Twila had no time for friends. Part of what she had enjoyed so much as a young child was the social aspect of directing others in her dramas. But all her lessons left her with almost no time to develop or sustain relationships.

Finally, in high school Twila called it quits on being responsible. She quit going to lessons, quit school and hung out all day with other drop-outs. She tried a few drugs but didn't like the way they made her feel. And after a while she also didn't like the way she felt hanging out at someone else's place every week.

So Twila decided to get a job that would allow her to make decent money, get her GED and have time to be with friends. She took a job as a waitress and immediately liked the social aspect of her work. Then she met a nice man in a mid-management position with a small firm. Before too long, they married. Together, they've been able to establish a pleasant, low-key life. Twila takes on small jobs that are not taxing. She occasionally models clothes, fills in at the local boutique, or waits tables in addition to caring for her house. She doesn't stay with anything for very long nor does she get very involved.

When asked if she has any creative interests, Twila's face tightens and she seems uncomfortable. She'll tell you "no" emphatically because creative activities take too much time. In her mind being creative means taking lessons. And that means having no time to enjoy life. It's hard to tell how long it will take for Twila to find that the creativity she enjoyed as a young child is still inside her and that it doesn't have to imprison her.

Perhaps saddest of all, Twila's parents do not understand what happened. They meant well. They were trying to support and help their daughter, of whom they were very proud. They didn't mean to hurt her. But they just didn't understand her true needs.

Recognizing Your Natural Creativity

You can begin to identify and recognize your own natural creativity by thinking back to your childhood. Whether or not you think of yourself as a creative person now, take a look at yourself when you were young. Like everyone else, you *are* creative. And you *can* reconnect with your creative roots to fuel your current life.

Think about your answers to the following questions. And be honest. There are no right or wrong answers—no answers that point directly toward or away from creativity. Remember to answer the questions only in relation to your childhood, not to the person you are now. The purpose is to discover the natural talents and gifts that you were blessed with in childhood.

1. What did you like to spend your time doing as a child? Include everything from structured activities to just hanging out. Be as specific as you can. Don't judge your answers. Just think back and be honest.

2. What games did you like to play, either alone or with other kids? Did

you make up your own games? Did you have a friend you particularly enjoyed playing with? Why? What did you do together?

3. When you were in a toy store as a child, which toys were you most attracted to? Or did you prefer to play with real-life things rather than toys? If so, what were those things?

4. What made you happy as a child? Remember times when you were happiest. What were you doing? How old were you? Did you continue to do these activities? If so, for how many weeks, months, or years? If you didn't continue those activities, what stopped you?

5. What made you feel satisfied?

6. When did you feel content?

7. What made your heart feel good?

8. What made you feel proud?

9. What kinds of problems did you solve as a child? What did you do to solve them? (And don't worry about whether or not the problems were considered creative problems.)

10. What could you not stop doing?

Now go back over your answers and notice incidents when you played with something or figured out a way to make your play more fun than it would have been if you'd followed the rules exactly. Did you improvise or make things up? What were you doing when you used your imagination?

What did you dream about with friends? Did you talk about your dreams with others? Did you try to make your dreams come true? Did you write about your dreams? Did you draw pictures about your dreams? Do you still have any of your writings or drawings or models of your dreams? Let yourself follow this line of thought now as you think back about childhood dreaming.

Notice how you felt when you engaged in different activities. Pay particular attention to when your heart sang. Think about the times when you didn't even want to stop what you were doing to go in for supper.

Then look at how your friends participated in those activities. Notice any differences between how you tackled problems, activities, and play time from the way the other kids did. Look for reflections of your unique approach to what you were doing.

Because being creative also means living a creative lifestyle (as opposed to having one specific easy-to-recognize talent) you may not have had one particular interest but may have had a creative flair when you were playing. Were you often making things up? Were you frequently the leader, making up games for a rainy day when there was nothing to do outside?

Do you remember a time when you were sick? As soon as you felt well enough to do something but still had to stay quiet, what did you like to do? How did you improvise when you didn't have the materials you needed to make something?

I want you to recognize the many ways in which you were creative as a child—and that includes doing things in your own way. To allow your creativity to show in this way, you needed to have been supported in your quest for independence. Were you always expected to follow the rules and color in the lines?

Individuality, improvisation, and uniqueness are all key words that indicate that you may have been doing things creatively. Change, differences, experimentation, and expansiveness are all signs that you were being creative.

Creativity for children comes out in many forms—playing with your food at the table or cutting your hair in a new and seemingly strange style. Even painting your body with bubbles in the bathtub or purposely putting your clothes on backwards may have been a way that you demonstrated your unique creative nature.

Yes, you were creative. I hope by now you recognize it, too.

Learning to Recognize Your Creative Potential as an Adult

You need to distinguish two kinds of creativity as an adult. The most commonly recognized type of creativity reflects a specific talent that is probably obvious to you and others. But another form of creativity is reflected in the broader form of living a creative lifestyle—meaning that you put together jobs, living arrangements, and relationships in new and creative ways. Though you may not have one single pronounced talent, everything you are involved with may reflect your creative touch.

If you do have a specific creative talent, you are likely to see it reflected in your work or hobby. The most obvious are artistic, musical, and expressive talents that showcase a specific skill, often one that you've worked hard to cultivate or perfect. Writing, composing, and public speaking are all examples of creative talents.

But there is so much more to creativity. You may be a creative building designer or problem solver working on anything from the design of new homes to the creation of computer software. Perhaps you are a creative thinker who conceptualizes new theories or programs. Maybe you have the insight to develop an effective environmental project or social program. You might be an auto mechanic who can fix just about anything. Maybe you invent make-shift tools when necessary to get the job done. Maybe you are a seamstress who adapts clothing designs to accommodate differences in body types, or a housewife who throws dinner parties that keep her guests talking for days. Maybe you have turned your creative skill into a job or career. Or maybe not. But either way, you are creative.

For example, consider Jacqueline. Jacqueline is a talented, accomplished playwright and director but has chosen to work in a civil-service job to provide the income and lifestyle she desires for her family. She knows that theater pay is low, work is sporadic, and time demands are high and inconvenient for raising children. When she looked at her whole situation, she decided she'd probably burn out quickly if she tried to force herself to write and work in the theater to earn a living. So instead she became involved in her local community theater as a hobby. She feels creatively satisfied and financially secure at the same time. Jacqueline's decision did not diminish her creativity. Rather, she feels it is protecting her creativity.

Willis does not have one particular outstanding talent. He likes to do many things—gardening, building outdoor furniture, sculpting, building rustic homes, writing books—and is fairly good at all of them, but he's never been able to pick one to pursue in depth. For as long as he can remember, Willis has loved to learn new things. He always finds an innovative way to accomplish new tasks. Recently, he went to a civic club meeting and, before he knew it, he created a fund-raiser to help overcome a budget shortfall. Earlier that day he figured out a way for his daughter to meet the demands of her school assignments and still join him on a field trip he thought she would enjoy. He also helped his wife figure out how to best utilize the laundry-room space so that she would have room to set up a sewing machine.

No matter what Willis is doing or where he is going, he leaves a path of modest innovation behind him. Even his lifestyle has followed that pattern. In school he majored in multi-disciplinary studies. He chose subjects that interested him and put them together in new ways, ways that highlighted connections between them that no one else had seen.

When he left school, he went into business for himself specifically to avoid having to do the same tasks or same job all the time. Also, he recognized that he had many interests and wanted to explore each of them in his own way, in his own time. So he contracted with people to do one type of job for a while, then shifted to another. It's not that he was irresponsible. He made sure he could pay his bills and that he didn't inconvenience others before changing projects.

Then Willis began to realize that several of his interests fit loosely together. From that realization he decided to create an outdoor-living business that allowed him to combine his interests. Sometimes he designed outdoor landscaping and built garden sculptures. Another time, he built a rustic home and the furniture that complimented the home.

Next, Willis created his own catalogues and built a model display area. When potential customers came to see his work, they would stay for quite a while because his display was so inviting. Willis often sat down with them, answering questions, sketching landscaping suggestions, and explaining how he worked.

One day, when someone asked to take his sketches home, Willis decided that he needed to write a book to share his sketches and explain his landscaping ideas. Since that time, one book has led to another. And only time will tell the many ways in which Willis will continue to enjoy and exhibit his creativity.

Living a creative lifestyle is not likely to bring you awards, nor will you be lauded by society as someone with an exceptional talent. The violinist, fashion designer, playwright, and choreographer might win the "creativity awards" from society. But you must know in your heart that your generalized creativity is valuable and innovative. You must ultimately be the judge of your creative endeavors.

Don't be fooled if you've not been discovered yet. It doesn't mean you're not creative. Creative people are often way ahead of their time and can see the broad picture long before others. Very creative people often lead frustrating lives waiting for others to catch up, so their work can be recognized or they can be understood. But what a waste of time to be waiting on others for that validation! Ultimately, you must be the final judge of your work. Lack of outside recognition does not mean that your work is any less than another's. Judge for yourself and decide whether or not you've done the best job you can do. Then look around and determine whether you can honestly see a place where your work fits in now. Assess whether or not you're ahead of the game. If you are, bide your time and watch for opportunities as society's interests shift. Twenty-five years down the road, the timing might be right for your work to be discovered.

CREATIVE POTENTIAL

Are you reading this book and wishing you were creative? Wishing you had accomplished something—anything—that you considered creative? Well, if you have those wishes you are creative, even if you haven't yet recognized that creativity inside yourself. We only desire what we have talent for in ourselves. You would not be wishing to be creative if you weren't creative already. That means your creativity may be in potential form, as opposed to realized form. But it is right there inside you.

If you cry or hurt inside, grieving that you are not the one being acknowledged for a creative act or performance, you are grieving the separation from your own potential. Maybe you don't believe in yourself. Or maybe you haven't been able to give yourself permission to be creative. But either way, you are cut off from the creative pursuits that you desire. You can change that by giving yourself permission to reconnect with your creativity, permission to use that creativity in any way you want.

When you hear yourself say, If only I'd done such-and-such, I could be doing what that person is doing now, you know that you have an unfulfilled potential lying in wait within you. Similarly, feelings of jealousy always come from feelings of inadequacy within ourselves. Wanting what someone else has—whether it's a relationship, a one-person show or a job creating innovative programs for the needy—only means that you are seeing something that you want but feel you aren't capable of achieving. So when you feel jealous about another's creative opportunities, know you're not a bad person. You're just a person who hasn't yet connected fully with your creative potential and found ways to manifest it.

When you find an urge or desire within yourself to create something, follow it as far as you can. I know that can be difficult sometimes. Fears about changing from a safe-feeling status quo may make it very hard to think about, much less plan, what you could do to resurrect your creativity. But your natural creativity, once reawakened, will not leave you alone. Its urging, like a sleeping giant aroused, will press you to find ways for its expression. You can fight it or try to ignore it. But your creativity will not go away.

So you might as well begin to enjoy it. Seek safe outlets that you can use to express it. Find other people who are interested in sharing creatively, and you will begin to harness a wonderful part of yourself.

If you're still not sure, or are afraid to let yourself believe, that you have creative potential, see if you can answer "yes" to any of these questions.

- Do you desire to be creative?
- Do you long to express yourself creatively?
- Do you admire people who are creative?
- Do you wish you had the time to do something you feel is creative?
- What do you daydream about doing? Is it creative?
- Would you like to do things differently on the job, at home or in other aspects of your life?
- Do you feel an urge sometimes to be free from having to just earn a living so that you could do what you really want to do?
- How would you spend your time if you had unlimited income without having to work for it? Would you spend your time being creative?

- What is your heart's desire? Is it creative?
- What do you feel you just have to do to be happy or feel successful? Is it creative?

"Yes" answers mean that your creative potential is alive and intact. Your job is to let it out. What a nice thing to do for yourself!

Remember. If you desire something, you cannot but have it as a part of yourself.

If you have desire, do you have talent? How sad to have to ask the question as I once did. But neither of us is bad for asking it. It just means that we have been separated from our natural creativity. We *can* reconnect. To the degree that you *want* to be creative, you *are*, in fact, creative.

You can find your own hidden creativity by listening to your deepest desires and allowing yourself to become fully aware of what you feel. That means feeling urges, desires, excitement, and sadness within yourself. Those feelings will lead you to what you desire and what you are separated from.

Each person has a full complement of skills within but, depending upon the style of ADD wiring with which you are endowed, your creativity will take different forms. If your form of ADD is are Outwardly Expressive, you will more than likely enjoy personally displaying your creativity through an expressive art form such as comedy, dance, or acting.

If you are Inwardly Directed ADD, you will tend to create art or crafts, design and invent things, or engage in creative thinking. Your creative productions may be used by others rather than be expressed by yourself. Because you are less likely to be interested in sales and marketing than your Outwardly Expressive counterparts, you may have a tougher time getting your work out. The key will be to have someone help you who can sell you and your productions.

If you are Highly Structured ADD, you may become very focused on one art form or creative endeavor. To be sure, you will tend to be perfectionistic in what you do. Precise, intricate creations are likely to be your venue. Depending on whether or not you also have some Outwardly Expressive ADD, you will have an easier or more difficult time getting your work out to the public. Again, the marketing and sales of creative work has little to do with the creative person's inclinations. Yet marketing does play a major role in your becoming known for your creativity, and your ability to use it successfully in your best interest.

Whether or not you ever become known for your creative endeavors, always remember this one thing—no one can ever take away your creative lifestyle.

It doesn't matter whether you work for a corporation or are self-employed, are displaying your talents openly or in private, or have a specific marketable talent or not. Everything you touch will carry your trademark, from the way you stack the dishwasher to the way you mow your lawn. Throughout your life, you will discover that you express your unique creative spirit over and over again. Your job is to keep your senses open and watch carefully for signs of that creative spirit. When you do, you'll see how wonderfully creative you really are.

chapter four

The ADD/Creativity Merger

A S YOU KNOW by now, there are many personality and learning conditions characteristic of ADD. Some seem negative, making some aspects of life more difficult for the person with ADD. Some seem positive, making certain situations easier for someone with ADD. Of course, by virtue of the name Attention Deficit *Disorder,* you are likely to consider yourself to have problems because you are ADD. Consequently, I'd like to start with a list of what are seen as negative ADD characteristics. But I will follow it with a list of the flip sides—the positive sides—of these same characteristics. By examining these lists, you will pick up the flavor of how ADD works within you, how it influences your behavior and shapes your perception of the world.

ADD: THE NEGATIVES AND THE POSITIVES

Here are some of the aspects typically associated with ADD that apply to people who demonstrate Outwardly Expressed ADD or Inwardly Directed ADD. They are described in a negative manner.

> Distractibility
> Poor concentration

Hypersensitivity
Impatience
Impulsivity
Hyperactivity or restlessness
Poor time management
Poor attention to detail
Difficulty breaking tasks into manageable bits
High risk taking
Wide mood swings
Procrastination
Temper
Reactivity
Daydreaming
Blaming
Getting stuck on projects

Here are some of the aspects that apply to people who demonstrate the Highly Structured form of ADD. They are described in negative terms also.

Excessive talking
Compulsive behavior
Difficulty creating a structure and unable to work without one
Difficulty recovering from change
Demanding
Over-organizing
Temper
Over-focusing
Very controlling
Rigid
Judgmental

Now let's look at the flip side. Here are some of the attributes of ADD described in positive terms for people with Outwardly Expressed or Inwardly Directed ADD.

Sensitive
Empathic
Deep feelings
Doing things in own way
Inventive

Unique perspective
Perceptually acute
Spontaneous
Fun-loving, fun to be around, playful
Humorous
Energetic, open, unsecretive
Eager for acceptance and willing to work for it
Responsive to positive reinforcement
Quick and intense, if he likes what he is doing
Looks past surface appearances to the core of people, situations, and issues
    Down to earth
Sees unique relationships between people and things
Cross-disciplinary and interdisciplinary
Likely to do things because he wants to, not because he should
Not likely to get in a rut or go stale
Original

Here are some of the aspects of Highly Structured ADD described in a positive way.

Appreciative of quality and willing to work for it
Well-organized
Leads forcefully
Intense when on a mission
Focuses for long periods
Holds high standards
Neat

CREATIVITY: THE NEGATIVES AND THE POSITIVES

Now let's take the same perspective in looking at creativity. First, let's look at some of the negative attributes that are often associated with creative people.

Unaccepting of or questions laws and rules
Cares little about cultural courtesies and standards
Doesn't much care what others think
Stubborn
Uncooperative
Resistant to authority

Feels others are wrong or out of step
Often doesn't like to join the crowd
Demanding
Assertive
Autocratic
May not do well in groups
Disorganized with "unimportant" matters
Careless
Sloppy
Self-centered
Intolerant
Impulsive
Impatient
Changes direction without apparent cause
Moody
Overly sensitive
Forgetful
Absent-minded
Inattentive
Spends time daydreaming
Overactive physically or mentally

Now let's take a look at the positive attributes associated with creative people.

Aware
Imaginative and original
Independent
Self-starting
Risk-taking
Energetic
Curious
Humorous
Attracted to novelty
Tolerant of disorder
Artistic
Open-minded
Perceptive
Intuitive
Spontaneous

ADD AND CREATIVITY: SOCIETY'S JUDGMENTS

I'm sure you are struck, as I am, by the similarities in the lists of negatives and positives for ADD and for creativity. The bottom line is that people who are creative often have many ADD attributes. That is not at all to say that creative people would necessarily be diagnosed as ADD. But they certainly share much in common with people who are ADD.

I've noted for some time that people who are ADD often are creative. They think creatively, do things creatively and independently, march to the beat of their own drum. However, creativity is not seen as a diagnosable condition—one found in the *Diagnostic and Statistical Manual* of the American Psychiatric Association. Consequently, no one knows how many people are creative, nor do we know how much their creativity gets in the way of their living up to their potential. And what would that potential be? If we are talking about one's potential as a linear-thinking, linear-oriented record-keeper in this culture, then creativity will definitely impede a person's ability to live up to that potential.

But our society generally is respectful of and makes allowances for the attributes of creativity. Consequently, the negative behaviors of a creative person are more likely to be excused, rather than judged. For example, people might say, "Oh, he acts that way because he's creative." Chances are, that statement would have been made with a smile or a laugh and without any negative judgment.

Unfortunately, those same allowances are not made for people who are ADD. They're also not often made for people whose creativity is revealed through a creative lifestyle as opposed to a particular highly visible talent.

Consider the person who works creatively, putting many different interests together. If that person happens to come up with a useable product or service, she is considered brilliant, a creative genius. But what happens to the person who is involved in many creative interests but isn't so good at interrelating them? Chances are, that's called job-hopping.

The majority of the problems attributed to ADD are the result of secondary problems that occur because our culture is becoming increasingly less user-friendly for people who are ADD. Unlike the unconventional traits of creative people with an obvious talent, ADD issues are not accommodated by society. Those differences are not honored.

For example, people who are ADD need to learn by doing. The apprenticeship model that has faded into the past served us well. But today most education is designed to teach people *about* something, through reading and lectures, rather than giving them hands-on experience. This poor fit between mainstream education and ADD learning styles can result in the development of low self-esteem, a less-than-satisfactory education, and trauma resulting from the ADD student's high level of sensitivity—hypersensitivity that is usually overlooked by the educator.

If these secondary problems are removed—in other words if people who are ADD are given an opportunity to learn in the ways that best suit them—the core attributes of ADD suddenly take on a new look: hypersensitivity becomes sensitivity that can be worked with in such a way that reactivity, oppositional behavior, and temper do not need to be much of a problem at all. Someone who is ADD can be taught organizational skills that fit well with an analog mind rather than to organize in a linear fashion. As a result, the attributes of ADD would be seen as positive rather than negative.

ADD and Creativity: What Do They Have in Common?

Let's look at the attributes of ADD and see specifically where they intersect with those of creativity. Although not all attributes of ADD are also characteristic of creativity, the following negatives seem to be applicable both to people with Outwardly Expressed ADD or Inwardly Directed ADD, and people who are creative. Such people are.

- distractible and have poor concentration when working on projects that are not of interest
- hypersensitive
- hyperactive or restless
- poor at time management
- likely to have difficulty paying attention to detail
- high risk-takers
- impatient, especially with routine mundane activities that take time and focus away from activities of interest
- likely to have wide mood swings
- likely to have a problem with temper control
- likely to be very reactive
- likely to be daydreamers

The negatives associated with people who have Highly Structure ADD are not usually shared by people who are very creative.

Next let's compare the positive attributes of ADD with those of creativity. The following characteristics of people who are Outwardly Expressive ADD or Inwardly Directed ADD also apply to creative people. These people are.

- sensitive
- empathic

59

- likely to feel deeply
- likely to do things their own way
- inventive
- likely to see things from a unique perspective
- perceptually acute
- spontaneous
- fun-loving, fun to be around and playful
- humorous
- energetic, open and not secretive
- quick and intense, if they like what they're doing
- likely to look past surface appearances to the core of people, situations, and issues
- likely to see unique relationships between people and things
- cross-disciplinary and interdisciplinary
- not likely to get in a rut or go stale
- original
- likely to do things because they want to do them, rather than do things because they should do them.

People who are Highly Structured ADD and people who are creative tend to be.

- appreciative of quality and willing to work for it
- forceful leaders
- intense when on a mission
- likely to focus for long periods of time on projects they enjoy
- likely to hold high standards

Now let's reverse the process. Let's look at the characteristics of creative people that could also be associated with ADD. First, let's list the more problematic characteristics. People who are creative and people who are ADD are often.

- stubborn
- uncooperative
- resistant to authority if it conflicts with an inner value
- demanding
- assertive
- autocratic
- likely to not do well in groups

- disorganized with "unimportant" matters
- careless
- sloppy
- self-centered
- intolerant
- impulsive
- impatient
- likely to change direction without apparent cause
- moody
- hypersensitive
- forgetful
- absent-minded
- likely to daydream and be inattentive
- overactive, physically or mentally

Finally, let's look at the positive attributes of creativity and see how many are also characteristic of ADD. People who are creative and people who are ADD are.

- aware and perceptive
- imaginative and original
- independent
- likely to be risk-takers
- energetic
- curious
- humorous
- attracted to novelty
- tolerant of disorder (with the exception of Highly Structured ADD people).
- artistic
- open-minded (with the exception of Highly Structured ADD people)
- perceptive
- intuitive
- spontaneous

Looking at these lists of amazing similarities, is it any wonder that it's often difficult to distinguish people who have an ADD style of brain wiring from people who are considered creative? In fact, the tremendous similarities between these two groups of people may indicate that the conditions of ADD and creativity share a similar neurobiochemical basis. I am not saying that *all* ADD people are creative nor that *all* creative people are ADD. I don't know that at this time.

Many questions will remain about the relationship between ADD and creativity until comparative reviews of both groups of people are undertaken in a systematic way. At this time, however, we can draw three main conclusions from observation: 1) A person who is ADD is also likely to be creative. 2) Many of the ways in which creative people cope with life would probably work well for people who are ADD. 3) There are probably many creative people who are wired in the ADD way but, because of their creative talents, have been excused for their linear learning handicaps or have found ways to be successful in life that use their talents and nullify much of the effect of ADD.

In thinking about yourself and your own situation, you must realize that neither being ADD nor being creative are mutually exclusive. Remember that there are many ways in which ADD can manifest itself and also many ways in which to be creative. At least three types of behaviors and personalities are currently being labeled as ADD. Creativity might be reflected in a specific talent or in an overall lifestyle.

Your best bet is to consider your options, let your heart lead you, and know that if you want to be creative, you are creative. If you like the ways successful people who are ADD live, then you, too, have within you what it takes to live a successful ADD life.

Enjoy either or both!

The ADD Mind vs. the Non-ADD Mind:
Setting and Reaching Goals

The ADD mind and the non-ADD mind work in very different ways. The most obvious of these differences is the way in which these two minds travel from point A to point B.

The non-ADD mind goes from point A to point B the straightest way possible. To the outside world, this looks like the most efficient way and, therefore, is considered to be the "best" way.

The ADD mind, on the other hand, takes detours. To the outside world these detours look unnecessary and off-track, and it's true that the person with the ADD mind might get to point B later than his non-ADD counterpart. However—and this is the key issue that is often missed by those who are judging the effectiveness of people with ADD—the person with ADD might reach point B in better shape to accomplish his goals than his non-ADD counterpart.

As examples, let's look at three scenarios. Think about each of the characters as you meet them. Why does each person do what he or she does? What are his or her goals? How does he or she want to live life?

Similarly, if you are ADD, give yourself permission to look at the value of how you do things—rather than automatically buying into the party line with regard to how you *should* do things. As someone who is ADD, your behavior is often judged by the standards of others, but as you read through these scenarios, consider that your personal life goals may be different from those of the people who are judging you.

First, let's meet Tom and Arthur. Tom and Arthur both live in Chicago and plan to drive to Florida to sell earthenware pots. Both have the same goal—to be a successful salesperson and make the best living he can.

Tom, who is not ADD, gets in his car in Chicago and drives straight to Florida using the shortest, quickest route possible. He feels good that he gets to Florida in record time and can begin selling his pots right away.

Arthur, who is ADD, starts out to do the same thing and also gets in his car in Chicago. But as he drives, Arthur begins to think about a friend who lives in Texas. The more he thinks about his friend, the more he wants to see him. So Arthur heads southwest. And as he's thinking about how good it will be to see his friend, he recalls that this friend has been experimenting with new, improved firing techniques for earthenware pots—techniques that make the pots more durable and better for cooking.

Granted, when Arthur first got the idea to turn to Texas, he didn't *consciously* remember that his friend's skills and interests could help him with his business goals. But one of the best-kept secrets regarding people with ADD has to do with their minds seeking reasonable, though often not immediately evident, reasons for changing direction. When an outsider determines that someone with ADD has gotten off track, the person making that judgment usually doesn't examine the situation in depth. For example, if someone had questioned Arthur, asking specifically, what he was thinking about when he made the turn, or to tell him about this friend Arthur he wanted to see, the sound reason for visiting that friend would become obvious. Of all of Arthur's friends around the country—and he has many—he thought of the one who had interests and skills that could eventually contribute to the fulfillment of his business goals. This kind of intuitive connection is often a part of an ADD person's life.

In the short run, getting to Florida as quickly as possible would seem to be the best way to reach that goal. But in the long run, it might or might not be. In any case, the quickest way is certainly not the only *sensible* way to get there.

People who are ADD tend to see a global picture. Consequently, they often work at bits and pieces of the total picture, seemingly at random, nudging each piece forward a little at a time. In the short run, it may seem that they're not making much headway. But in the long run, they may just end up with the whole pie, rather than only one quick piece.

So, Arthur goes to Texas and talks to his friend about the new techniques for making earthenware pots more durable. He immediately sees implications and possibilities for the market he serves. He leaves Texas with new ideas, more opportunities for reaching his ultimate business goals, and a heart filled with warm friendship.

Heading east to Florida, he notices that his uncle, who lives in Alabama, isn't too far out of his way. Arthur recalls his uncle has many business contacts in Florida and throughout the South. Though, initially, he only thought of tapping his uncle's contacts in Florida, he realizes that there is no reason to only work the Florida market. So he deviates one more time from his initial plan and stops in Alabama to get advice and direction from his uncle.

By telling his uncle what he is doing, Arthur will probably be opening a channel that will continue to produce ideas and leads for many years. His uncle, flattered that Arthur has sought his advice and pleased that he could help a young person get going, will most likely take it upon himself to do what he can to help Arthur out. The result will probably mean a lot more business, some direct and some indirect, for years to come. So this detour also produces a wonderful support system for Arthur.

As he speaks to his uncle, Arthur learns the value of casual networking rather than spending a lot of time cold calling. By taking the time to develop relationships with people, he discovers that they truly want to join his team and provide ongoing support that yields results.

To be sure, Arthur arrives in Florida several days later than Tom. And Tom has already sold a lot of pots by that time. But by the end of the month Arthur has set up an ongoing network that yields a continuous and improved product line and potential buyers. Tom, on the other hand, has to return to Chicago to get another load of the same pots and soon begins to saturate the market in Florida. He plans to move on and open another market when this one dries up, but that means starting over from scratch.

As you can see, Tom met his short-term goal more quickly than Arthur. But Arthur matched, or surpassed, Tom's long-term goal by working in a different way—one that fits him better.

Now let's consider Heather and Maria, both of whom design furniture and enjoy that business. Heather, who is not ADD, has one goal—to sell the most furniture she possibly can and make the most money she can, so that she can retire with a sense of security. That is the one goal she is always working toward.

Heather also likes people and enjoys the contacts she makes selling her designs. In addition to her financial goal, she judges her success as a person by how many contacts she has and how many friends she makes.

Maria, who is ADD, also designs furniture and wants to be successful. But her goal is different than Heather's and the way she measures success is different. Maria loves to create new designs. She gets easily bored refining old designs and selling the same ones over and over. So her goal is to create a new design for every piece of furniture she sells. She also loves to make new contacts but tends to spend time with people whom she enjoys, rather than people who can necessarily help her out with her business.

Maria doesn't much think of the future. She's very involved with whatever she is doing at the moment and fails to make long-term plans of any kind, though she does have dreams. But somehow, her plans for her dreams rarely get carefully thought out, much less implemented. She measures a good month by how many creative designs she's made, how pleasurable her relationships have been and whether or not she can pay her bills.

Measured by Heather's standards, Maria might not appear as successful as Heather. But measured by her own standards, by what's important to *her* in life — Maria is very successful. Their paths and styles of living are just different.

Finally, I'd like to introduce you to Ginger. Ginger, who is ADD and very creative, was raised with fairly traditional values. Her parents, having gone through the depression of the 1930s, encouraged her to train for a profession, which she did. But Ginger, despite her considerable formal education, wanted to live a creative lifestyle. She wanted to be responsible and not depend on others, but she also had desires in her heart that she felt she had to honor. And she wanted to earn her living by implementing those desires.

Even her educational choices didn't make much sense to others. At first they didn't make sense to her. For example, she majored in sociology and psychology as an undergraduate. Then she decided to become a counselor, so she could help others as well as understand herself. But when an opportunity arose to earn a master's degree in anthropology, she thought the subject sounded exciting, and she went that route. Ginger hadn't given up on the idea of becoming a counselor, but despite others telling her to get a master's degree in psychology, she went forward with her own plans. All of her papers and independent studies in anthropology emphasized the psychological aspect of what she was studying.

As she was completing her course work for a doctorate in anthropology, she noticed a fellowship program that sought to train predoctoral anthropology students in clinical methods so they could do clinically sound field work. Ginger jumped at the chance, won the fellowship and gained the very clinical skills that she'd wanted to achieve in the first place. Then she was drawn to the community mental-health movement that wed individual psychology with social and cultural environments. Needless to say, Ginger did particularly well because of her diverse background.

Years later, Ginger achieved a high level of success as a clinician, author, and speaker. A lot of her success was due to the diversity of her training, which led her to see things in just a little different way than the average professional. She often said that the best teacher she ever had was anthropology because it taught her to look at the world through others' eyes and not be limited by the value system and perspective of the world in which she was raised. She knew that her way of doing things was not the only way and that others often felt as strongly about their way as she did about hers.

Ginger's professional training and career path were unique. She lived and learned in a creative way that honored her interests. To be sure, she occasionally was passed over for jobs that required a more traditional background. But by going into business for herself, she discovered that she was often hired as a consultant or speaker to those same groups that wouldn't have hired her on staff. So she ended up having her cake and eating it, too.

Ginger felt she had no alternative but to live from her heart, moving through life in a way that felt right to her. She simply couldn't bear to do things that didn't fit her or to do things that sapped her creative nature. Instead, she found ways to get what she wanted, honoring herself. And Ginger didn't mind her circuitous route. The journey was one that held her interest, rather than imprisoned her.

Though Ginger did not consistently make as much money, or accrue retirement benefits, as some of her peers, she did make enough to live a very comfortable life. She still never knows if one of her ideas will hit the jackpot, making her better off financially than her peers, but Ginger wouldn't trade her way of doing things for any amount of money. She loves her life, and lives it day by day—rather than living for retirement. Ginger did a good job for herself and others by following her desires and respecting the way in which she is wired.

CREATIVE VS. NON-CREATIVE THINKING

When your creative mind clicks into operation, you will tend to see the overview of the situation in which you are interested. You may have a vision that your heart wants to fulfill. You are likely to have a creative thought and see the whole thought completed in your mind.

For example, suppose Walt Disney conceptualized a theme park in his mind. He would have imagined lots of activities and experiences for park visitors to participate in, and he might have realized that it could become similar to a year-round world's fair. First he had the idea of the theme park. Then he probably saw in his mind the completed theme park up and running. His mind might be spinning in many directions at once, thinking about the kinds of rides, how they would look, and how happy they would make people feel.

The problem for many people—and I don't know whether Mr. Disney had this problem or not—comes in planning the millions of details that it takes to bring such a vision into reality: budgets, site planning, contracts, logistics, schedules, materials, and workmanship, to name only a few. When the creative idea comes into the mind of someone who is ADD, all these middle planning steps tend to be missing. The planning, logistics, and organizational pieces often call upon the exact skills that are compromised because of ADD. Even for the person who is creative and not ADD, his mind is likely to spend more time spinning creative ideas than doing the nuts-and-bolts work necessary to get a project or idea up and running. Creativity is simply different from some parts of administration and implementation.

For example, consider Sandra. Sandra is a clothes designer whose creativity includes the styles and decorative aspects of the clothes. She also creates clothes specifically for people with figure flaws and for people who have physical difficulties getting in and out of clothing. Sandra is truly a creative genius.

Sandra's problem comes once the designs and prototypes are completed, the fabric is chosen, and samples are made. Setting up and managing a manufacturing facility, along with obtaining the capital to go into full-fledged production, requires skills that Sandra just doesn't have. Recognizing that her talents are in the creative area, not the administrative areas, Sandra enlists the help of others. Unfortunately, she does not necessarily make wise employee choices. She also fails to keep an eye on her interests—preferring instead to design more styles, seek unusual fabrics, or figure out how to solve a style-show dilemma.

Sandra's mind just doesn't think about practical details. Even when she tries, she doesn't ask the right questions and doesn't have a tangible criteria upon which to base her decisions. Somewhat distractible, she agrees to whatever anyone tells her if they speak in an authoritative manner.

A creative idea in the hands of a linear thinker is wonderful because the middle step—the nuts and bolts needed to implement the creative idea—is in place. The only problem comes in relation to the possibility of getting bogged down in details and not reaching the end vision. A linear thinker either takes a long time to get things done, or a very short time, with limitations to the creative expansiveness of the original vision.

For example, Harrison, an engineer, had a dynamite idea for redesigning a water-treatment system in the plant where he worked. He showed his plans to his boss. His boss liked what he saw and told Harrison to go ahead and work up a complete plan and implementation program. Harrison was delighted and figured that he might even win an award for his design.

But the problem came when Harrison's creativity pressed him to redesign every joint and turn in the plumbing. He spent a lot of time researching materials. He focused for long periods on every aspect of his project.

Finally, his boss told him to either finish the implementation plan or scrap the whole idea. There wasn't anything wrong with Harrison's idea, but the combination of his hyper-focus on details and his creativity caused him to fail to get the job done in a timely manner.

Faced with his boss's ultimatum, Harrison did finish, but he felt cheated. He wanted to apply his creative mind to every facet of what he was doing and resented having to just get things done.

Pat, on the other hand, thinks creatively at times but very clearly shifts gears once he identifies his goal. Pat is a contractor who builds many homes on speculation. When he commits to build a house, his mind works in two ways. Initially, he is in a creative mode. He plays with ideas, designs, and materials, and allows his mind to run free. But once he's decided it's time to build, he chooses his style, materials, and design and puts other ideas aside to use later for the building of other houses. From that point on, Pat's mind functions in a linear mode unless he hits an obstacle that does not allow him to follow a preset plan. Then he returns to his creative mind-set and redesigns that particular aspect, switching back to his linear mind-set to complete the building.

Pat's creative mind is expansive and he lets it go for broke. But when he begins to implement the plan that his creative mind has devised, he's all business, and he focuses on staying on track. Pat's ability to consciously decide how he wants to function is a great asset for him.

It's important that you understand that there are no right or wrong paths to follow here. But if you can become aware of how the creative mind works and how the ADD mind works, you can better understand your own successes and difficulties. The way someone's mind works can influence the outcome of the project he undertakes. I just want you to be aware of that.

COMPARISON OF GOALS: PEOPLE WITH ADD AND PEOPLE FOLLOWING THEIR CREATIVITY

As we've seen in the examples above, two people can be doing the same thing but be working toward very different goals. For people who are ADD and creative people, the process is more important than the end goal. The scenery along the road traveled may be at least as important as getting to the destination. That does not mean that creative and ADD people don't have goals or that they don't keep those goals in mind. They do.

Remember Arthur. While on his way to selling earthenware pots, he developed an entirely new business-networking structure. He tracked down someone who had developed a whole new method of glazing pots. In the end he did just as much, if not more, business than his non-ADD counterpart. It's just that he reached his goal by different means.

Being ADD, Arthur's major focus—what's important to him—is different from someone who only focuses on the end goal, blocking out everything else so as not to get distracted.

People who are ADD cannot *not* see the many stimuli around them. And creative people cannot *not* create. That's just how their minds work. For both types of people, every perception is multi-faceted with many implications and choices. That's just how things are!

How Does Your ADD Impact Your Creativity?

Being both ADD and creative can provide you with a wonderfully interesting life. But it can also create some problems that non-ADD creative people don't face.

For example, consider Gary. Gary has looked at the world through a creative filter from the earliest time he could remember. He loves to paint and draw, carve and create sculptures of all kinds. And he always demonstrates a lot of skill in the areas in which he's interested.

But Gary is also ADD, and he never did well in school. He managed to get through, but his self-esteem suffered because he is brighter than his grades and amount of education would indicate. He also was told that he couldn't make a living doing art work and to get a "real" job.

So at graduation from high school, Gary went to work in a manufacturing business. In all of his off hours he pursued his hobbies, as he called his artistic interests. But he never really tried to market his work. He would do things for friends and family and had a lot of work stored in the corners of his yard. When someone wanted to buy a piece of his work, he usually declined or underpriced it.

Gary just couldn't see that he could possibly create anything that had value. In his mind he was a school failure and, therefore, a failure in life. His creative work suffered from this deeply held belief—a belief that stemmed from his ADD difficulties.

Rosaria is a woman I know who suffers from organizational difficulties—and I do mean suffers. She has so many projects going at once that she never really gets much meaningful work done on any one project. She loves to dance and teaches dance classes, but because she doesn't market herself consistently, her classes often dwindle to only a few students over time. She also has a marketing company with some very good ideas for clients. But, because of the clients she chooses, Rosaria either doesn't get paid at all or is paid only modestly.

For example, she recently staged and marketed a dance review and a performing arts piece, both of which showcased the work of other artists. Rosaria worked hard and the shows were successful. But when it came time to divide the profits, she was somehow left out. She had failed to carve out a specific reimbursement plan for herself ahead of time.

Over a period of six months I saw Rosaria write several columns for her local newspaper, talk about starting a magazine of her own, meet with two other people about starting a magazine and check into a computer-based communications project. One time she created a particular product that seemed to have potential for success. But she was unable to figure out how to market it. In desperation, she signed up for a small-business class. But she left at the end of the first night when they said she needed to start by making out a business plan. She told them, "Get real! If I could do that I wouldn't need your class."

Rosaria wasn't trying to be rude. She just was completely frustrated. The ADD part of her felt overwhelmed and found it impossible to figure out where to start writing a business plan. Although the teacher had clearly outlined the steps involved, Rosaria couldn't understand what was being said. She felt panicky and quit.

The bottom line is that Rosaria is a very creative person who cannot maintain her focus of attention on any one path long enough to make any significant headway. She is unable to deal with the business end of her enterprises, and that keeps her from becoming financially successful. And she has not found anyone to work with who will not take advantage of her.

If Rosaria could find the *right* people to work with her, she could use her ADD to her advantage. With her many interests she would do well to team with a different person for each interest.

For example, let's look first at her dance classes. Even though she has many creative marketing ideas, she is not consistent enough to keep her classes full. But Rosaria would do better not having to spend her time trying to do what is so hard for her. Instead, she would do well to focus on her creative, artistic abilities so she can contribute from her areas of strength.

Rosaria needs to simplify her business by hiring a good assistant: a secretary, agent, or money manager. Or she could make a trade with someone to run that aspect of her business in exchange for marketing services, dance lessons, or whatever else they can agree on. This same person could help her focus on a couple of projects at a time so she doesn't spread herself too thin. And he or she could negotiate deals for Rosaria to make sure she is fairly compensated for any work she undertakes.

But Rosaria's ADD makes her want to do things in her own way. And that means she has real trouble cooperating at times and is less than willing to follow directions. Consequently, her "assistant" would need to include Rosaria in the designing of the assistance Rosaria needs. That's asking a lot of an assistant—but it's important.

With the details of their relationship worked out and with the business aspects of her work under control, Rosaria would be free to enjoy her creative energies. Her impulsivity, properly channeled and supported by a teammate, would be turned into spontaneity. Her high energy level would provide her with the ability to implement several projects at once, thus keeping her from getting bored and bogged down.

In other words, with the proper teammate Rosaria could use her ADD to become the success that her creativity demands.

How Does Creativity Impact ADD?

As we saw above, Rosaria's life was complicated by being both creative and ADD. Her ADD works both for and against her creativity. Now let's look at Rosaria's situation from a different perspective and ask the question, How does her creativity impact her ADD? The answer again is both negative and positive.

Rosaria's creativity could work against her by providing her with the ability to create imaginative "lies" in an attempt to hide the fact that she didn't get her work assignment done on time—the one she'd promised her assistant she'd finish in time for a major deadline that could mean big bucks. Then, having procrastinated until the last minute, Rosaria would not be prepared for either the flu bug that might seek her out or the family emergency that could disrupt her ability to work. Her problem results from not having left extra time for unplanned interruptions.

Feeling irresponsible and guilty, both feelings she'd endured for years as a student, Rosaria might invent a phenomenal lie to tell her assistant. And lying probably would have worked before for her because of her creativity. Teachers, parents, and college professors had probably bought in on her stories for years. If she hadn't been so creative in dreaming up the stories much earlier, she would have had to face the inevitable results of putting things off until the last minute. Now, untrained to be truthful, she might lose a major job, a considerable amount of money, and the respect of those who had been trying so hard to help her. Thus her creativity would have gotten in the way of her implementing her creative abilities.

The whole trick for Rosaria is to figure out how to use her ADD in creative ways and her creativity as an asset to her ADD. Rosaria must learn to utilize her creative talents constructively while learning to get her ADD under control. Depending on her particular situation, medication might be one positive step toward helping Rosaria focus on work more effectively. But medication alone will not retrain the bad habits she's learned.

Her job is to learn the coping skills she needs to help control her problems with organization, lying, follow-through, and impulsivity. First and foremost, Rosaria must learn to tell the truth. Then she must commit to do the best she can to follow projects through to the end, not committing to projects that she realistically cannot get done. Management of her impulsivity comes next as she learns what triggers her impulsive actions and finds alternative ways to get her needs met. Finally, she can be helped to find simple organizational methods that work for her.

With her ADD under control, Rosaria can begin to unleash the positive aspects of her creativity and her ADD. With a framework in place, she can generate ideas and create parts of projects guided by the outline created by her assistant. She will know when to ask for help, which frees her to go for broke in her desire to make her dreams a reality. Hand in hand, her creativity and her ADD can work in unison, supporting one another.

Evaluating Your ADD/Creativity

I ask you now to look at yourself. You know about being ADD. You know what you can do to manage it by making up for the inadequacies created because of your style of brain wiring. You have committed to improving your skills one by one; those that are within your capability to improve. And you've agreed to seek assistance for those that you do not have control over.

Now check out the creative side of yourself. Affirm your talents whether you've gained recognition for them or not. Acknowledge the importance of living a creative lifestyle. Consider how important it is for you to live with your creativity showing. Affirm your willingness to use your creativity to its fullest.

Take your time. And don't make any commitments to creativity that don't feel right to you. But whatever you do decide, know that is the right way for you at this time. It may or may not be the right way for the rest of your life. But you are dealing with the present now.

Next, decide whether you want to see your ADD and your creativity as assets or liabilities. It's your decision! Yes, I'm placing the responsibility on you. That's the bad news. The good news is that taking that responsibility also opens all kinds of possibilities for you. I am suggesting that, in fact, you can choose to see your ADD and creativity in a positive, even wonderful light.

I know that your ADD has made things difficult at times for you over the years. And you might think that choosing to see it as something positive sounds like a joke, even a cruel joke. But I assure you that you do have that choice to make, and it can make a tremendous difference in your life.

Of course, you can continue to view your ADD, your creativity, and yourself in a negative light. If you do choose to take that negative viewpoint, I suggest that you are probably comparing yourself to others so that you come up feeling "less than." If you do, I'd ask you what your criteria for judgment are. Do you consider yourself "less" because you earn less money, have less schooling, less fame, fewer friends?

If you are comparing yourself with someone else, I'd ask you to consider making a different comparison. Instead, consider comparing your current situation to the talents you have within yourself. If you are not working up to your *own* potential, then I can understand your wanting to do better. If, however, your comparison is to some standard outside of yourself, I'd wonder where and from whom you learned that point of view. None of us can be like anyone else. You can and need to be only like *yourself*.

Consider Mike, a professional photographer. At thirty-four, Mike began to wonder about himself. He wondered whether or not he was successful. He wondered if he should be doing more with his life than he had been. He was concerned that he wasn't making much money—certainly not in comparison to many of his contemporaries. Although he had been artistically satisfied during the early years of his career, he no longer felt that sense of satisfaction after photographing too many sinks and vegetables for advertising clients. On top of everything else, he wasn't making much money, in part because of his ADD problems that showed up in the area of billing and collections. True, Mike had learned to live on a shoestring. But he wondered if he'd ever be able to make enough money to support a family or even to get ahead himself.

All these feelings came to a head when Mike attended his high school reunion. Comparisons smacked him in the face. Many of his old buddies were much better off than he was financially. No one seemed particularly impressed with the fact that he'd managed to earn a living as a photographer for more than fifteen years and was well respected in his field. His work, good enough to win him the opportunity to teach high school students throughout the country, was of little value to those who didn't understand his creative lifestyle.

Mike came home from the reunion and shared his feelings with his parents, who assured him that he was doing fine. But he still had doubts. When he talked to other creative friends, they just shrugged, having run up against those same feelings themselves.

Then Mike talked to himself. He tried to picture himself doing something else for a living, so that he would appear to be more in the mainstream. But every time he thought about that, he began to feel very depressed. And he really couldn't think of any "real" job that he thought he could tolerate or that he had any hope of succeeding in.

Next he turned his attention to his finances, and that proved to be a real struggle. He felt overwhelmed and completely incompetent to manage them. The organization of such details was far beyond him.

His reverie led him into remembering how hard school had been. He knew he was bright but that he hadn't done well in school. Mike just never managed to get the classwork quite right, though he wanted to and he tried. He made good friends and fit in socially, but academically, he felt his life was a disaster.

Close to spiraling down into depression, Mike called a friend who said, "Get a grip! Remember who you are and what your life is about."

So with this new approach to looking at himself, he began to remember his assets. He realized he was a wonderful person. He recognized that he was a very good photographer, even exceptional at those times when he was photographing a subject that pleased his heart. He recalled that he *had* managed to succeed, though maybe not at the financial level of some of his professional peers.

As his thinking took this more positive direction, his heart began to swell, and he remembered why he liked living a creative life. It was then that the light bulb went on in his head. He suddenly realized that he'd been comparing himself with others, rather than looking at what he was doing with the talents and interests he possessed. He realized that measuring himself by the amount of money he made just was not an important standard for him to meet. Doing a job that he felt good about—that's what was important to him.

So Mike decided that he'd photographed enough sinks and vegetables for a while, and he put his creative energies into finding jobs in which he could reflect the human condition through his photographs. As soon as he took that step, he felt much better about himself. He felt that he was doing something worthwhile, and he felt confident that he would make enough money to be comfortable. But he also realized that making lots of extra money was not his issue. Doing what he loved from his heart *was* his issue.

Mike weathered his introspective storm and came out accepting and loving his gifts of ADD and creativity.

CREATIVITY AS A SURVIVAL SKILL

As you know, being ADD in this culture can be tough because so much of what is expected and valued doesn't fit you. Yet as I've been saying, you are valuable. I promise you.

If you allow yourself to become immersed in all the things you don't do well because you're wired in an ADD fashion, you will, in fact, see yourself as "disordered." But I'd like to suggest an alternative.

If you will take the natural creativity that so often accompanies ADD and use it to your advantage, you will have found a resource that will stand you in good stead. Actually it can save your life—or, at least, your happiness.

Creativity can be a survival skill for ADD people. It has been for me in terms of the joy I get from writing, doing artistic projects, and solving problems creatively. Even as you or I have to deal with monthly bills, stacks of paper, boring learning situations, insensitive people who don't understand our levels of sensitivity or a host of other ADD-related situations, we can find respite in our creativity. We can use it to make life rewarding, as a payoff for doing the yucky things that don't come easily. Or we can even use it to create a life that honors our creativity and our ADD.

Just as designers have created their own styles of jeans the last couple of decades, so, too, can you create a "designer life." You are capable of designing your life any way you want, based on how you feel about yourself and what you enjoy doing. Your quality of life will be determined by how you choose to spend your time and the attitudes you bring to each day.

ADD and creativity can be seen as a curse or blessing. How do *you* want to see these issues? The choice really is yours to make. To be sure, you will pay the price for whatever choice you make, but that's not all bad. Payment of a price simply means that you have opted for behavior that is comfortable for you. Although it may be a behavior that runs counter to what is usually thought of as correct you get to determine your own response and then go forward.

The only time I feel resentful or depressed about paying prices is when I've bought into something that doesn't fit me. If I maintain my integrity, stay honest with myself, respect my gifts, and live an authentic life that fits me, I never mind paying my bills.

You, too, can live this way.

Design your own life. Listen to your heart, then use your mind to implement your choices. Then you are on your way.

So, how do *you* want to create *your* life?

chapter five

Where Did Your Creativity Go?

WE DON'T DO THAT."
   Did you ever hear that sentence from your parents when you were a child? Maybe you were putting your finger in a glass of soda to see if you could feel the bubbles. Or maybe you were drawing with crayons on the sidewalk to see if the color lasted longer than chalk. Whatever you were experimenting with, that phrase let you know that it was not okay to pursue that line of creative thought.

Parents never mean to purposely take away their child's creativity. But it happens often because of thoughtless habits that parents learned when they were young themselves. Most of us act that way, myself included, until we wake up and listen to what we are saying or see what we are doing to our children.

Jill remembers walking by her refrigerator one particular day when she was in sixth grade, and noticing that she could see a shadowy reflection of herself in the refrigerator door. Her science teacher had been speaking just that week about the fact that only very smooth surfaces could reflect light back to the viewer. So Jill ran her fingers up and down the refrigerator door to test it for smoothness. She remembers comparing that in her mind to the way a mirror would feel. Just as she was moving her fingers all over the door, her father came into the kitchen.

"How many times have you been told to keep your hands off the furniture?"

he yelled. "You'll get your fingerprints all over everything." Jill tried to explain about her science teacher and reflections, but he wouldn't listen.

I know Jill is a creative person, but she doesn't see herself that way. Why? Because she learned in her kitchen, and other places, that pursuing creative activities is not the way to live life. Obviously that one incident did not steal her belief in her creativity. But I'm sure the tone in her home conveyed the same message repeatedly.

Jill's dad is not a bad guy. He simply didn't realize the many implications of his daughter running her fingers over the refrigerator. Many parents in our culture are very concerned about neatness and cleanliness. Much is made of doing chores, which usually means cleaning house and taking care of one's property. Somehow there is a cultural belief that if a person and the things in her life are neat and clean, she is a good person who will be valued and better protected from bad things happening. It's all a matter of trying to gain control over life.

Many parents have fairly rigid parameters by which they judge the world and their child's behavior. Even if the behavior isn't hurting anyone and is fairly harmless that particular behavior might not fit into the parent's ideas of what is and is not acceptable.

Not long ago, I noticed a three-year-old trying to teach himself how to tie his shoes. He tried pulling the strings this way and that way. He didn't become discouraged when they kept falling loose. He just kept trying. Though very intent, he wasn't frustrated, and he didn't ask anyone for help. He enjoyed experimenting with the laces. When his mother walked by, she saw what he was doing and said, "I don't have time now, but as soon as I finish what I'm doing I'll show you how to tie your laces the right way."

When she returned a few minutes later, ready to show her son the "right" way to ties his shoe laces, he shook his head "no," jumped up and ran into the other room to do something else.

His mother shook her head, too, not understanding why he didn't want her help. "I don't know what gets into him," she said later to a friend. "When I try to show him how to do something, he gets up and leaves."

What his mother didn't understand was that three-year-olds are emotionally focused on trying to do anything and everything that comes within their reach — by *themselves*. They are interested in the *process* of doing things, not the outcome or what adults would see as the goal of their project. This three-year-old's urge to try to do everything by himself carries the seeds of later creativity and a sense of competence that the child can do anything he tries to do.

By trying to show her son the "right" way to tie his shoelaces, this child's mother missed a teachable moment. What needed to be taught was not how to tie his laces so they'd stay tied, but that he is a person who can feel competent and creative. She might have said, "I see you are trying lots of ways to tie your laces. Wow, you are so creative (or skillful, or a good experimenter). If you want me to show you another way (not the "right" way) to do it, I'd be happy to. Just ask me."

If you haven't been encouraging your child's creativity in this way, don't feel too bad. I didn't always encourage my children's creativity when they were little, either. I didn't fully understand the importance of it at that time. But I do know now what needs to be said in order to help our children stay connected to their creativity, and I know that one of the ways in which creativity is closed off is a short, subtle comment such as: "We don't do it that way."

I do realize how hard it can be when a parent has fifty million things to do in a day. Some days are so chaotic that you just really want to get things done quickly. That's when you probably don't feel you have the patience to let your child experiment with six different ways to get his shoes on. You might want to fight that chaotic feeling by having the things around you neat and in order. Unfortunately, that's probably just when your preschooler will decide it's time to start taking things apart. So take a deep breath—because I have to tell you that taking things apart is an important part of creativity in childhood.

Sal and Lonnie were neighbors. Both boys loved to take things apart. Sal's mom didn't like it when he dismantled the vacuum cleaner, tried to take all the knobs off everything and pried his toys apart. She made him stop, scolded him, and told him to go read a book.

Lonnie's mom laughed when he did much the same thing and gave him a tool box with tools. She set limits by telling him clearly which household items he could and could not take apart. She also often asked him to help her because he did such a good job taking things apart. As he got older, Lonnie also learned to put things back together. Before long, Lonnie was building things on his own, inventing all sorts of contraptions, and well on his way to living a creative life.

In contrast, Sal was afraid to try to do anything on his own. Even in high school lab courses, he wanted to follow the procedures exactly so he would do the experiment right. Though Sal had the same initial creative urges that Lonnie had, his were driven underground. He did not see himself as a creative person and felt very uncomfortable in situations that were not rigidly structured.

Sal's mom wanted the best for her son. She wanted him to do things right, just as she'd been trained. She had worked hard for her money and didn't want things broken. She had a great deal of respect for certain objects and wanted to instill this same respect in her son.

What Sal's mom didn't realize was that she could set limits on Sal's experimentation—instead of keeping him from it all together—so he would learn that respect while still being given the freedom to follow his innate interest in seeing how things work. She didn't mean for Sal to become fearful, even though she was afraid of trying things. She had no idea that her fears stemmed from much the same training—training that teaches that something bad will happen unless she does things in exactly the same way she was raised. She quit experimenting and so did Sal.

This is one of the ways that creativity is shut down.

WE DON'T SAY THAT WORD

Children tend to be very creative in their development of language. Even older children, especially those who are ADD, will use words that aren't necessarily real, but they do convey to a listener the exact intent of what needs to be communicated.

Callie, for example, asked her mom for a "door opener" instead of for a "key." It was fortunate for her creativity that Callie's mom responded with, "What a creative way to describe a key. I understand perfectly."

Haven't many of us gone into a hardware store and described a tool or piece of hardware by its function rather than its name? That's creative—using the function of what is wanted when the name is not known.

But what if Callie's mom had been concerned that her daughter didn't know the word for "key" and missed an opportunity to see both how creative her child was and how her child's mind processed information. Such functional descriptions, commonly used by people with ADD, serve the purpose of identifying an object and also demonstrate the brain's analog processing style. The reward of allowing words to be used this way is the enhancement of creativity.

Parents don't need to be concerned that those of us who are ADD will arrive at school or in the workplace with our own special vocabulary, unable to communicate with others. Of course, we do learn labels—the ones used by everyone else. But we also keep our ability to use descriptive language when we don't know, or can't recall, a label. So, in a sense, we have two language systems.

How wonderful! That means that one system does not need to be thrown out for the other to be learned. But because you may have been told as a child, that's not the right word to use, you may have been cheated out of an opportunity to encourage development of your creative side.

People who are not necessarily ADD, but who think strategically, also create language in a different way that enhances their ability to keep their creativity alive and well. For example, when Grant was about three years old he invented a couple of words that made a lot of sense to his parents. They joined him by starting to use the words, too. Here's what happened.

When a person makes a contraction of the words "you are not," he says, "you aren't." The words "he is not" become "he isn't." So, following the same form and rules, Grant decided that the contraction of "I am not" would be "I amn't."

Grant's parents recognized the mental process that he went through to arrive at the newly crafted contraction and they used it, too. They weren't afraid that he'd go to school in a couple of years using it, since he'd have lots of opportunities to hear the accepted way of saying "I'm not." And that's exactly what happened.

But if Grant's parents had been less aware of the mental process going on or more concerned about Grant learning correct grammar at age three, they would have corrected him and told him that his way was wrong. As a result of that correction, Grant might have felt that his natural, creative mental process was wrong. The resulting doubt in himself and his abilities would have been big enemies of his creativity.

OVER-SOCIALIZATION

In the name of socialization, a lot of creativity is dammed up, or even buried, for people in this culture. Often inadvertently, the teaching of manners inhibits the development of creativity when we are young. For example, did you hear, "Don't touch things," "Don't stare," or "What's wrong with you, don't you know how to behave?" Yet, rather than being discourteous, you were probably only curious and your curiosity got the best of you. The result of those restrictive statements was the inhibition of your natural creativity.

Does that mean that children, or anyone else for that matter, should be allowed to ravage, break, or disregard other people's property or to act in discourteous ways toward others? Of course not. But the trick is to not throw out the baby with the bath water.

Respect of other people's property is essential. So when a child reaches for an object in a store or someone else's house, a parent might say, "I know how curious you are, but we can't touch anything that isn't ours without permission. Let's ask if it's okay to touch it." What's important about this reaction is that it validates the child's inquisitiveness and does not say he did something wrong. However, it also teaches respect for the property of others. This child remains curious—an essential component of creativity.

But what if that child's parent had hit him in public, yelled at him, or said, "I don't know what's wrong with you. I can't take you anywhere without your getting into trouble." Do those phrases make your stomach knot up just a bit? Is it still hard for you to let yourself go and explore materials, techniques, or ideas? Or can you laugh about how you touch and handle things you come in contact with? Your response is an indicator of how well you have weathered one of the roads that leads to creativity.

Even if your parents disciplined you positively by distracting you or gently teaching you how to behave, your creativity could have been affected if your curiosity was not reinforced and redirected. Fortunately, though, your mental health would have escaped damage.

Many years ago, one of my children, age five at that time, walked up to a woman in a wheelchair and said, "How come you're in that chair instead of walking?"

Does that sound familiar? Many children ask that question at some time. The first thoughts that raced through my mind at that time were based on the way I had been raised. I thought, Oh, no, what will the woman think of me and my child.? Will her feelings be hurt?

Fortunately, being as ADD as I am, I process a lot of thoughts simultaneously and very quickly. So I was able to move on to another batch of thoughts before I responded to my son's comment. That next batch was based on what I had learned about children. I thought, How wonderfully inquisitive my child is. I wonder how the woman feels about his question. What can I do to help the situation and be sure that everyone feels okay?

So I took my son's hand and said to him, "You're really curious about this chair and the way this woman gets around, aren't you?" He nodded with a serious but expectant look on his face.

Then I quickly looked at the woman to see what her reaction was. If it had been stern or unhappy looking, I would have excused us and turned to my son and said, "Let's go talk about wheelchairs and how people get around." Then I would have steered him aside, and we would have had a conversation about the subject. I'd have also told him that not all people are comfortable talking about being in a wheelchair, and it would be a good idea to ask me his questions first. I would have told him I wanted him to have all the answers he'd like and would talk with him anytime about anything.

As it turned out, I could tell by the woman's smile that she would be delighted to talk with an inquisitive little boy. We went closer so my son could touch the big silver wheels. She explained about her chair and told him how long she'd been in it. She told him that it took some getting used to but that she was sure glad to have it since her legs didn't work anymore.

Then, she turned to me and said how wonderful it was to have a conversation with someone out in public. She mentioned that people often ignored her just because she was in the wheelchair, and even asked her husband questions that she needed to answer rather than asking her directly. She also recalled with delight how her children had been curious when they were young and how it had stood them in good stead as adults who were still curious, creative people.

What a wonderful encounter. I've never forgotten this grand lady! Nor have I forgotten my son's curiosity.

TIME FOR LESSONS

The most typical block to the development of a child's creativity, especially an ADD child, is the assumption that because the child likes to do something creative, it means lessons are in order.

I call this the "piano lesson syndrome." It goes like this: A parent notices that her child is musically inclined and likes to play around with the piano. The parent immediately assumes this means that 1) The child should have music lessons, and 2) The child will want to take music lessons. This parent really is trying to tune into the child's creativity. But the attempt often backfires for one of two reasons—either the lessons don't fit the child's learning style or he doesn't really want structured lessons. He just wants to explore.

Either way, the lessons have the effect of shutting down creativity, sometimes for years. I shared my own "piano lesson syndrome" experience with you in chapter 1. In my case, I had liked the idea of lessons. I wanted to learn to play the piano. But what I needed were fear-free lessons that helped me learn the way I learn.

In retrospect I would have done better if the teacher had been able to use a multisensory approach with me. Instead of giving me a piece of music to learn, the teacher might have sung the song to me first, had me hum it with her, danced with me, beat the rhythm out on a the piano bench with my fingers or drawn a picture about the music as well as have me take the music with me to also learn to play. Since I'd have already known the sound and rhythm of the music and would have enjoyed being involved with it, I would have had a good feeling about the piece. Also, I would have learned it faster, which would have cut down on practice time.

Then, because of my restlessness, the teacher could have broken the music down into small segments and suggested that I only practice a couple of phrases for a short time, maybe just five or ten minutes. Maybe she could have suggested that one of my parents join me to practice part of the time so that I would have some help focusing my attention.

Finally, she would have needed to tell me that making mistakes is a wonderful part of learning. She could have told me that she makes mistakes even now and surely made a lot of mistakes as a child learning to play the piano. She could have reassured me that one day I'd learn to play without mistakes, but this was not the time. If I appeared anxious, she might have told me she wanted me to make some mistakes so she'd have something to do to help me in my lesson. And the next time I made a mistake, she would have congratulated me saying, "Good for you. You're learning."

But this type of learning experience isn't the one most of us have. Instead, well-meaning parents spend money to help us develop an interest without realizing that our creativity can be jeopardized.

I'm not saying that all lessons are bad. I am saying that care must be taken—whether the student is a child or an adult—to make sure that taking lessons doesn't interfere with creativity and expressiveness.

If you are currently taking lessons to get a better grasp on some creative activity that you like and you're turning off, don't automatically assume that you are no longer interested in the material. Check to be sure it's not the way in which you are being taught that is turning you off. You might do better to explore more on your own or find a different teacher. I'll tell you my story about changing teachers in chapter 9. It can work wonders.

TESTING THE TESTS

School and teachers have a tremendous influence on us. The schoolteachers you had as a child, most of whom were trained in noncreative environments, shaped how you now feel about your creativity. Think about how much time you spent with your teachers, how much you looked up to them and how much you learned from them about what is acceptable behavior.

Again, though no one planned that your creativity should be undermined in the school learning environment, several factors greatly compromised its continued health. The grading process is the first culprit.

The whole process of marking children's answers right or wrong is a very hurtful, noncreative process. Think about it this way: An answer is usually considered either right or wrong. Learning is forced to focus on getting a preset answer that allows neither for alternative ways to accomplish things nor for alternative outcomes. Your getting a particular right answer is then used to prove that you have learned something—which may or may not be the case. And that rigid, limited piece of information will only be useful to you in the future if you are confronted with a very similar situation that requires the same answer. You haven't really learned how to think for yourself.

Instead, suppose a teacher were to respond to one of your answers with, "Okay, let's see how you came to your answer." Then the teacher could either find out where you got off track, or see how you came up with an inventive solution that makes perfect sense. You might even have reordered or invented something new. At least you would have been given an opportunity to learn to think.

If you were not blessed with this kind of open approach to learning, you would not have had opportunities to give explanations of what you did and why. The result of that can be an adult who is fearful of new situations—fearful because he might not know the one right way to act in the face of this new situation, or the one right answer to solve the new problem. He wouldn't have had much confidence or practice being an inquisitive explorer.

The next culprit is testing. This concept sounds like a tongue-twister, but think it through carefully with me: Most tests test what the person who makes up the test believes. Think about it: Right answers are the *test-maker's* right answers. Wrong answers are the answers the *test-maker* considers wrong. This is particularly true of fill-in-the-blank, multiple choice, and true/false tests. Even essay tests may require a singular thought process to prove that the test-taker knows about the subject being tested in a particular way.

So students cram for tests second-guessing what they think is going to be on the test. And a lot of time is spent figuring out what the teacher wants to hear and in what form, in other words "psyching" out the teacher. That type of "studying" is very limiting and definitely is not conducive to creativity.

I recall taking a state licensing exam many years ago in the field of counseling. I was exhausted when I left the testing room. That's because I knew exactly which answers were considered right, but I had different ideas about mental health and the origins of specific behaviors. So to pass the test, I had to put aside my own thinking and creative work and regurgitate what was expected.

But think about what it would be like if the focus of the test were on the student justifying his way of thinking. How exciting it would have been to have been able to set forth my own theories and show how I arrived at the results that I considered right.

For example, consider a licensing exam given twenty years ago. If you were asked how long ADD lasts, the correct answer at that time would have been, "until puberty." If you'd answered, "a lifetime," you would have been marked wrong based on the generally accepted concepts of that time. You would have been marked wrong—but your answer actually would have been right.

Suppose the question had been reframed like this: "Hyperactivity is less apparent in the lives of some adults who are ADD than in others. How might you explain this?" Then your answer might be graded based on your views of hyperactivity when it's used positively. You would have had the opportunity to mention how most of the top sales people of the country use their ADD to their advantage. You could then have earned a good grade.

I can also imagine that someone might take a totally different approach and still create a logical, consistent response based on his knowledge of the literature and his own creative thinking. Perhaps a totally creative answer would evolve from another person's different experience. How grand! I wouldn't even need to agree, but we could have a great discussion from our individual perspectives.

The whole point here is that tests tend to squelch creativity most of the time. If you believe that traditional tests do accurately measure knowledge and intelligence, then you probably have had your creativity limited. Consider rethinking what tests really prove. Maybe they only prove whether or not you agree with a particular perspective that has been labeled acceptable.

THE ROLE OF BOUNDARIES

Creativity cannot exist within hard boundaries, within a system of strict delineation between areas of thought. In fact, creativity tears down boundaries, brings elements together across boundary lines. Isn't that exactly what being creative is—putting things together in new ways? Creativity often reflects the process of how things are experienced and expressed, rather than details and steps contained within limits.

As I noted earlier, people who have Outwardly Expressed or Inwardly Directed ADD tend not to live within the confines of boundaries, limits, and details. If they do have boundaries in their lives, they have different ones than non-ADD people. Yet in our culture, acceptable boundaries are very clearly set forth. Rules, regulations, and beliefs reflect these tight linear boundaries.

For example, consider what happens when children are presented with coloring books and must color within the lines, or when they are criticized for coloring things unrealistically. A purple and pink pumpkin might bring a comment such as, "Oh, no, pumpkins aren't purple or pink. Pumpkins are orange with green vines." The creativity of the child is restricted because the child crossed a boundary—whether it was a physical line on a page or the line between fantasy and reality.

Another way to understand the rigidity of boundaries in our society is to consider the diagnosis of ADD. Let's look at the paths of three people: a licensed psychologist, a teacher, and a neighbor down the street.

The psychologist has studied psychology according to guidelines set forth in academia and passed state licensing exams in order to practice psychology. Because of these credentials, the psychologist is allowed to diagnose and "treat" ADD—regardless of how much she actually knows about ADD. She might never have studied ADD in depth, had a long-term relationship of any kind with someone who is ADD, and might not even remember much about it from school. But our culture says this person is the one to diagnose ADD.

The teacher, certified to teach, is not allowed to diagnose or "treat" the person who is ADD, even though she may be very familiar with the signs of ADD and know more about practical ways to help someone with ADD than the psychologist. The teacher can, however, be hired by a school system to teach certain specific skills to the person who is ADD. That's because our culture has labeled her a teacher. So, teaching is what she is allowed to do.

The neighbor down the street can neither diagnose, treat, nor be hired to teach someone who is ADD, at least not in state-licensed facilities, even though he may know more about ADD than either the teacher or the psychologist. This neighbor might be ADD himself. He might have raised two successful children who are ADD, and he might have hundreds of ideas about ADD and how to benefit from the ADD style of thinking. But he is a neighbor—not a psychologist or a teacher. So his opinion on ADD isn't valued.

This compartmentalization is the result of living in a linear culture that has strict boundaries identifying what is acceptable and allowable.

In a less linear culture with fewer rigid boundaries, things would be handled differently. In that type of culture people probably wouldn't be categorized as ADD in the first place. But if someone were considered to have a problem, that person would probably be helped by someone who had first hand experience with the issue. That might be a teacher, a person in the community known for her wisdom, a neighbor or a family member who had demonstrated a talent for working with the specific difficulty in question. No one would consider arbitrarily denying a community member the right to help if that person had the skill. In our culture, our clearly drawn boundaries tend to do just that.

Creatively speaking, boundaries inhibit and limit what *may* or *may not* be done—regardless of whether it *can* or *cannot* be done. Boundaries are often thought of as protections. Sometimes that's true. But more often they are used for the purpose of control. They usually restrict people instead of protect them.

WHERE DOES CREATIVITY GO?

Is it any wonder that a lot of the natural creativity with which you were born went underground? It may even seem as if it went completely away. You might even believe that you are not creative and never were.

Though I recognize that not everyone has the same amount or type of creativity, I do firmly believe that everyone has some creativity, though it might be hidden, and you can tap into as you wish.

As soon as I say that, I can hear some people countering with, "Well, I don't know. I sure don't feel creative, though I'd like to be." In response I promise you that to whatever degree you would *like* to be creative, you are creative.

I also know that you may need to retrieve the creativity that was set aside during your earlier life. To accomplish that, you'll need to think back and identify the specific ways in which your creativity was squelched.

Ask yourself the questions listed below—and pay attention to how the questions make you feel and what they make you think about. If you'd like, you can make some notes about what happens inside of you when you read through these questions.

You don't have to rush through this exercise. Spend as much time as you like on each question and be sure to keep track of your feelings. And remember—there are no right or wrong answers to these questions. They are simply included here as a tool for you to use in your effort to identify the path your creativity might have taken as a child.

1. Did you hear, "We don't do that?" Think of an example when you were exploring or trying something out and were stopped. Maybe you were even scolded or scowled at. Perhaps your mom or dad only told you to stop whatever it was you were doing, without an explanation.

2. Was there a time when you were trying to learn to do something, and an adult came along and showed you the "right way?" How did you feel?

3. Were you the kind of kid who liked to take things apart? Do your parents still tell stories about how hard it was to teach you to keep your hands off things?

4. Maybe you remember liking to try to do things when you were quite young, but then quit. Do you know why?

5. Do you recall playing with words, or does someone in your family tell stories about how you made words up? Were you corrected so that you would have "correct" language skills?

6. Were you a very "good" little boy or girl? Could your mom or dad take you anywhere?

7. Do you remember being reprimanded for your behavior, especially in relation to other people or when you were away from home or around other people?

8. Were you given lessons in anything, such as music or art? How did you feel about them? Were you scared or tense? Did you hate them, or did

you like them? Did the lessons make you want to do more of the activity? Or did you burn out, lose interest, or get bored after awhile?

9. How was school for you? Did you feel as if you were learning and able to be creative with that learning? Were you allowed to make a lot of mistakes, or were you being corrected frequently?

10. How did you do in test situations? How much time did you spend studying for tests rather than studying to learn about the subject?

11. Do you prefer to stay within strict or solid boundaries? Do you dislike or even hate rigid guidelines? Were you exposed to, and expected to stay within, boundaries, even though you would have preferred not to have them?

Look back over your notes now. As you answered each of these questions, how did you feel? By examining your answers carefully, you will find where you hid your creativity.

It could be that you had been very creative at one time, but stopped liking your creative activity—for any number of reasons—and so quit doing it. Or, like me, you may have continued to do the creative activity—but in secret, skulking around out of sight, hiding your productions in filing cabinets and storerooms. Maybe you found your cognitive mind lecturing you about how you need "to prepare for life" and must put away the playthings of childhood.

Now you can see how you learned to not trust yourself, your instincts and intuition, and why you put your natural creativity in hiding.

GRIEVING YOUR LOST CREATIVITY

The result of this hiding of your creativity could be that you have gone through a separation process from your creativity over time. You probably didn't intend to separate from your creativity, but you did, nevertheless, for your own survival. In most cases no one else purposely tried to take away your creativity. It happened because we live in a culture that doesn't value or accommodate creativity very much. Whenever you separate from something, you grieve. You and I would have grieved our separation from our creativity just as we would grieve the loss of a friend.

But the good news in this case is that your creativity isn't really gone forever. It is still there, and you can get it back. But I know it can feel like it is gone forever. That's why you grieve.

To understand how that grief might have affected you, let's look at the five stages of the grief process.

The first stage is denial. You know you're experiencing denial when you feel confusion, don't seem to care, or never think about something that previously was a part of your life. You may declare that creativity isn't really important anyway. Or that creativity is for childhood. Or that people who are creative can't do anything else in life. Maybe you just feel upset and confused when you try to think about creativity. All of these are indicators that you have unfinished emotional business with regard to your creativity and that you are probably still experiencing denial.

Anger is the second stage of the grief process. Anger is a cover-up emotion that protects your vulnerable feelings—feelings of helplessness, hopelessness, fear, or frustration. If you take a peek under the anger you feel about your creativity, you'll probably find one of your more sensitive feelings. Go about this process slowly. Let yourself grieve the loss that your anger has been protecting you from feeling.

Many creative programs in this country have been cut, and the explanation is usually something like a lack of funding, or that the programs are just a waste of time and money, just frills. When you hear these statements, notice if the person speaking them sounds angry. If he does, he is probably in this second phase of his own grief process—trying to stay as far away as possible from his vulnerable feelings about his loss of creativity.

This explains why some people have such strong negative reactions to creative endeavors. They have those strong outward reactions because they are not dealing with their own inner grief over being separated from their own creative natures.

The third stage of the grief reaction is bargaining or the "what if . . ." stage. It is characterized by attempts to second guess ourselves in order to fend off our sense of loss. So you might find yourself saying, Well, when I retire, I'll do something creative. Or you might think, that if only you had inherited enough money, won the lottery, or made a killing in the stock market, you'd be able to do what you really want to do. Maybe if only you could roll the clock back, you could prevent what happened.

Feeling guilty is another aspect of this second-guessing stage. It's the one I'm personally most familiar with. I continued to do some creative work but paid for my actions with feelings of guilt. Those guilt feelings were my psyche's attempt to change something that I didn't want to happen. Guilt makes us feel as if we have control when we really don't. By feeling guilty, I was saying, that I really shouldn't be doing this, but I can't help myself. So I'll experience guilt as an attempt to pay for being out of control. Maybe next time the guilt will steer me away from doing the creative thing so I can be more practical. The only problem is that it never works.

The fourth stage of the grief reaction is depression. You know you are getting close to accepting the loss of connection to your creativity when you feel depression. Being down in the dumps, hurting, and feeling depressed slow us down and keep us from doing things.

Being separated from creativity is the source of depression for many, many people. I have come to believe that it is one of the reasons so many people live lives of slow death as their creative potential goes uncultivated and unattended. After all, creativity brings life and sunshine into our daily existence. All work and no creativity makes any of us very dull and depressed.

Normally, the fifth stage of the grief reaction is acceptance of the loss. What is wonderful here is that you don't have to accept the loss if you don't want to — because the loss is only a perceived loss. Unlike the death of a loved one or even the loss of a job or opportunity, your creativity is not irrevocably separated from you. It didn't disappear. It just went into hiding. You have the power to reconnect with your creativity, to give yourself permission to utilize your creativity, and to value that aspect of yourself.

Now that you know why your creativity went into hiding and where it has gone, you have the opportunity to reprogram your beliefs so that you can reconnect with that side of your true nature. You can include creativity into your life to any extent that you want.

After all, you are no longer a child who is dependent on others for approval. You can think for yourself and take responsibility to live the kind of life you want. You have choices to make, and that means you have power. You have the power to make a decision to keep your creativity tabled, or decide to honor your creativity by letting it show.

If you choose the latter you can

- choose how and in what situations you want your creativity to show
- set your own limits on it
- give yourself permission to be the creative person you were always meant to be
- live a life that is centered around your creativity

Respect yourself for handling your creativity yourself, bringing it under *your* control rather than allowing it to be junked because of other people's attitudes.

Regardless of what you do, enjoy the decisions you make. You are a creative person naturally, and now you can be captain of your own creative ship.

chapter**six**

Creativity and Sensitivity

AS ANYONE ever told you to stop being so sensitive? How about this one: "Stop wearing your feelings on your sleeve?" Chances are you've heard them both, because if you're ADD and creative, you're probably a very sensitive person, also.

Sensitivity is an integral part of creativity. You might think of it as the life blood that feeds the body of your creativity. Without sensitivity—awareness of what is going on around you and in you—you do not have the raw material needed to create anything, whether that creation is an idea, an object, or an action. The more sensitive you are to your surroundings, the more aware you will be. And, therefore, the more you can tap into your creative capacity.

Regardless of whether or not you are ADD, sensitivity and creativity walk hand in hand. When you add ADD to the mix, you automatically have a heightened sensitivity to the common five senses of touch, taste, smell, sight, and sound, as well as a greater sense of intuition—a kind of inner sensitivity that feels what others are feeling and knows or senses what is happening at many levels in a situation. Having a heightened sensitivity to others also means you can often tell what people are thinking, their motives and intents. Even when you deny or don't realize your true feelings, as an ADD person you are likely to know the truth behind the facade.

Being ADD and sensitive also means that you are likely to get your own feelings hurt more often than non-ADD people. Because of your heightened awareness, you will feel everything around you intensely because your filter—your ability to keep stimuli away—is thinner than average. This is just the way you are. You didn't choose to be very sensitive any more than people who sunburn easily choose to have sensitive skin. It's just the way you are made. It is very important for you to understand that and accept yourself as you are.

I bet there have been times when you wished you weren't so sensitive. I know there have been for me—even though I consider my sensitivity to be one of my greatest gifts.

The bottom line is that it just plain hurts to be very sensitive. For me it means that when someone else hurts, I hurt, too. It means that I have to spend three or four days recuperating emotionally from having seen a film about the Holocaust, for example. And that's an improvement. When I was younger, such a film might have affected me for weeks, or even months.

What non-ADD people don't understand is that those of us who are ADD don't have a choice about our sensitivity. We are sensitive—and that's just the way we are. Our increased sensitivity is probably one of the least-recognized and least understood aspects of our ADD.

Creative people have more permission to be sensitive than those labeled ADD. It's part of the privilege that comes with being seen as different when the end result—some creative product or expression—is respected or accepted by others. Without this acceptance, your sensitivity may be seen as a problem rather than just the way things are.

But your sensitivity is simply an integral part of who you are and what you do. This section will help you appreciate your sensitivity for the contribution it makes to your identity and your creativity. You'll also find out how to protect yourself from some of the hurt that it can attract.

TWO TYPES OF SENSITIVITY

Being sensitive means that you are open to stimuli: the sights, sounds, tastes, smells, touch, feelings, and actions of what is around you. It also means that you are open to learning from what you take in. You will tend to recombine those stimuli into new creations. First your perceptions will change and then your actions as well as your perspectives, beliefs, and ultimately your reality, all based on your sensitivity to the stimuli you absorb from around yourself.

To illustrate this concept, let's look at two people who would react very differently to the same situation.

Suppose Jenny and Tobie both went to the grand opening of a local builders' supply store. As Jenny walked in, she immediately noticed the colored balloons decorating the entryway. She was very excited by the fuchsia-colored balloon and made a mental note to find out where she could get similar balloons for a benefit she was planning. She noticed that the light filtering through the balloons cast wonderfully colored reflections on the shelves of merchandise. She decided she would try to capture those tones in painting when she got home.

As Jenny walked up and down the aisles, she noticed and enjoyed the smells of the freshly cut cedar, pine, and oak. The hum of three electric saws cutting through different densities of wood sounded like an orchestra to her. The sounds made her feet want to dance as she walked.

Just then, she overheard a man complain about the store not carrying a particular product he wanted. She quickly looked up to see the reaction of the store clerk. He was listening stoically to the man's complaint. Jenny could feel their tension running through her body. She felt sorry for both the man who was disappointed and for the clerk who seemed helpless to do anything about the situation.

As she turned down another aisle, some noisy children ran past her. Although they were very loud, they were obviously having a lot of fun. Though their yelling hurt her ears a bit, their horseplay made her laugh as she remembered that she and her brother had done the very same thing not that many years ago. "Kids keep being kids," she thought.

By the time Jenny left the store, she had twenty ideas for projects she wanted to do. She had also solved a couple of problems that had been on her mind for a while. Seeing the fuchsia balloons had given her one idea about decorations for the fundraiser she was working on. She'd also seen some plywood cutouts, which reminded her that she could make silhouetted figures for the event she was planning that symbolically respresented the organization.

All in all, it had been a red-letter day for Jenny. New ideas, solutions to problems, and an all-around vital, fulfilling time spent at the store's opening. As she left, she felt happy but also exhausted. All that stimulation made her feel like she'd been working for twenty-four hours straight—that's how much she'd taken in.

While Jennifer was in the store, Tobie walked in. He noticed that the store was very crowded. As he passed by the balloons, he thought about getting one for his daughter who had stayed at home and decided he'd get it on the way out. He wondered how much inventory they had and whether he'd be able to order supplies that they didn't carry.

When Tobie passed by the man with the complaint, he thought about how hard it is to meet everyone's needs and wondered what kind of customer-service department the store had. Tobie watched the men talking. He was curious to see how the situation would come out, but he didn't feel much of anything for either person.

As Tobie headed out of the store, he had a pretty good sense of what the store carried and where he could find what he might want in the future. He remembered to pick up a balloon for his daughter and headed for his car, checking to see the quickest and best way out of the parking lot.

Jenny and Tobie had been in the same situation at the same time. But they each learned and absorbed different information from the experience. Jenny was physically tired from all the stress she had absorbed in the store. But her openness to the experience left her with many creative ideas and information about where she might find supplies. To Tobie the experience had been more concrete and simple—it was about a new place to buy supplies, and that was all it was.

In addition to being sensitive to stimuli, people who are sensitive are also very sensitive to judgment and criticism. It is this second type of sensitivity that tends to cause a lot of problems for people.

Whether or not you are ADD, if you create something, you are opening yourself up to the world. A very special part of you—your ideas and skills—are reflected in your creation. That makes you vulnerable. Unless you want to create something alone in your room and never have anyone see it, you are exposing your creative production and, consequently, making yourself vulnerable.

Making your production available for others to see instantly opens you to criticism. At least, that's how viewers look at creative production, whether they know you or not. Once a product or idea is made public, everyone sees it as fair game for judgment. And most of the time rather than saying, "I like it," or "I dislike it," the person will say, "It's good," or "The artist *shouldn't* have used those colors together."

You might think creative people would get used to that kind of criticism, but they don't. Instead, they usually feel hurt—over and over again. Most creative people learn to fake it, avoid it, or strike back. But the truth is that it just plain hurts to be critiqued, criticized, and evaluated. Yet, that seems to be the standard for the culture in which we live. Unless you lose your sensitivity—which also means you blunt your creativity—you are not likely to feel any better about receiving that criticism ten years from now than you do now. You'll just show your reactions differently.

The core of the inner, most vulnerable part of yourself is responsible for what you create. Now that the term "inner child" has been introduced into our vocabulary, I might say that it's the core of your inner child that you are sharing. Just as exposing your own babies to the world brings out a lot of protectiveness in you, so too does bringing out your inner child's creations. That's a good thing. I want you to protect those creations.

I've often wondered how someone can assume that they have some magical standard within themselves that allows them to evaluate another person's work. To be sure, there are cultural standards that, by definition, more people adhere to than not. But creativity means going beyond cultural standards to something new. That is why creative people are so often ahead of their time. They might be overlooked or poorly evaluated until years after first unveiling their productions.

Sometimes, too, a product that is marketed uniquely or more extensively is considered creative. But perhaps it is simply an old product marketed in a new form. That may be creative marketing, but it does not necessarily reflect a creative product.

It's important for you to realize that because criticism is generally nonconstructive, and even unkind, asking someone to get used to it, is not reasonable. If you feel bad when your work is criticized, that's a normal and reasonable reaction.

What a wonderful world it would be if we each pointed out what we *liked* about each other's creations and simply did not point out what we didn't like. Or if we at least took responsibility for the fact that it is we who don't like it, which is very different than saying the work itself is flawed.

One of the reasons we have so much "authoritative" criticism is that our culture clearly values the finished product more than the creative process. Creativity is often seen as superfluous.

ADD and Sensitivity to Stimuli

Extreme sensitivity to stimuli is an attribute of ADD, whether or not you see yourself as creative. It doesn't matter whether or not you have creative talents or live a creative lifestyle; if you are ADD you will be very, very sensitive.

Often, professionals working with ADD thought that children who were diagnosed ADD were insensitive. But the behavior thought to show insensitivity was actually the result of an extremely sensitive child learning very early in life to self-protect—to self-protect automatically. Even by birth, the sensory system of an ADD fetus has been barraged by stimuli—stimuli felt many times more keenly than by a non-ADD fetus.

Within the first six months of life the booming, buzzing confusion of the world around all infants can feel like a massive attack to a baby who feels, senses, sees, hears, tastes, and smells everything acutely. The seeming insensitivity is the result of the child metaphorically barricading himself behind a stone wall.

Sometimes the child learns quickly to self-protect by opposing the onslaught of stimuli. These children are called oppositional-defiant and have been thought to be insensitive. In reality they are so sensitive that they must react to try to protect their sensitive inner cores.

For people who are ADD, sensitivity can be a great and wonderful asset. But it can also be very, very painful. For example, consider Thomas. Thomas, a musician, enjoys his sensitivity. He loves lyrical music and knows he hears nuances others miss. He is a sensitive husband who responds to his wife with finesse, knowing when she wants him to be gentle, when playful, and when raucous. He reads his students well, too. In general, he enjoys adjusting his actions to fit the needs of the other person in a relationship. That's not to say he ignores his own needs. He doesn't. He's equally sensitive to his own inner urgings and gives himself plenty of opportunities to get what he needs. All in all, Thomas likes and utilizes his sensitivity to his advantage.

R. J., on the other hand, experiences a lot of pain because of his sensitivity — and he always has. He was raised in a verbally abusive family where his parents constantly told him how he should act and what he should feel. His parents often told him he was too sensitive, and his dad made an occupation of teaching him to be tough. R. J. married a woman who is quite insensitive. She is repeating the pattern he experienced growing up.

Though R. J. wanted to work with animals and be out of doors, he felt he had no choice but to do what his dad told him to do. So he joined the armed services and volunteered to go wherever the most action was — to prove to his father that he was tough. The result was a bad case of post-traumatic stress disorder along with drug and alcohol abuse. R. J. simply couldn't throw off what he was exposed to at home and on the front. He absorbed the pain around him and felt wounded, unable to get relief from his emotional pain except when he used chemicals — and that relief didn't last long.

Those of us who are ADD are so sensitive that we often have to protect ourselves from stimuli, and simplify what we are exposed to, if we want to remain emotionally intact. We don't need to be overly stimulated. In fact, it's a good idea to learn how to self-protect against it.

So, if you are in a very stimulating environment, you will need to be sure to take some time out for yourself. Meditation, music, a soothing bath, a body massage, or just being outside, away from the city can help. Make certain that your peace-seeking is a part of your daily routine, not something you do only when you get sick or overwhelmed. Why wait that long?

If you're involved in creative work, you may also need to self-protect — especially if you are taking lessons related to your creativity. Often teachers and well-meaning friends or colleagues feel they need to stimulate your creativity. But if you're ADD, chances are you have all the stimulation you need. For example, I've often heard non-ADD people say that they like to go window-shopping in malls to get ideas. But that sounds awful to me. If I did that, my mind would spin off in a million different directions, and I would feel awful. I don't need any more ideas or stimulation. If you feel the same way, you'll need to learn to self-protect.

Each form of ADD causes different reactions to stimuli, and each person self-protects based on his or her primary type of ADD.

People who reflect the Outwardly Expressed form of ADD tend to react openly. That's called acting out what you feel. This type of person is likely to become very hyperactive, tell jokes, spring into action, talk excitedly and begin to do ten things at once. Some people with this type of ADD simply tell it the way it is when a lot is going on.

Barb, a primarily Outwardly Expressed ADD person, went to Alaska for the first time. She had the opportunity to spend several days doing whatever she wanted. She jumped into lots of sightseeing, and became a whirlwind of activity. If she was with a group, they would never go as fast as Barb wanted to go. Barb would be shouting back to the group, "Come on, come on. You should see this. Wow. It's great. Hurry up."

While seeing the sights, she simultaneously utilized any creative talents she had. She took a sketch pad with her wherever she went, madly sketching scene after scene. Camera in hand, she clicked away constantly and make hourly entries in her journal. Stimulated by all the newness and all there was to do, she tried everything, and generally went nonstop until every bit of her energy ran out and she "crashed."

By the time Barb was ready to leave Alaska, she had a whole list of new people to keep in touch with. She created many new projects to pursue, dreamed up ideas for several new businesses, outlined a series of books in her mind, and decided to keep traveling—Scandinavia, Tibet, Nigeria—the farther from the familiarity of home the better.

Barb's problem came when fatigue crept up unrecognized. She became grouchy, argumentative, and used alcohol and drugs to try to calm down. She lost touch with the needs of others around her even when they clearly communicated their needs to her. It's not that she's self-centered. It's just that she gets caught up in all the new stimulation and forgets to rest. She doesn't mean to hurt anyone.

The other problem Barb faced is that all her potential creations required planning and organization. How, when, and where was she going to implement them? Her mind became confused as she jumped first in one direction, then in another. Soon she felt so overwhelmed that she could no longer manage effectively. At that point, she blamed anyone who was around—even though they had little, if anything, to do with her problem.

On the other hand, Larry, an Inwardly Directed ADD artist, had a different reaction from Barbara's. His ADD shows itself in restlessness, constant fidgeting, and daydreaming. Rather than acting out when he arrived in Alaska, he moved more slowly, trying this and that. Not very focused, Larry wandered somewhat aimlessly and began to daydream. When he saw his first glacier, he stared at its beauty. He began to think about how a glacier is made, how he could re-create its beauty so he could carry the experience with him, and what it must have felt like to be one of the first men to ever set sight on such a magnificent creation of nature. He became absorbed in his fantasy.

When Larry was in a group, he did not want to keep up with the faster pace of the others. He is easily overwhelmed and as a result slows down or even shuts down, wanting to completely stop. He would be quite content to linger, going at his own pace, but others may press him to see it all.

Larry absorbed the tones and feelings of what he was seeing. Rather than frenetically sketching or planning, he doodled, sketched a few lines, jotted an idea or two down in his notebook. Though his thoughts may be as complex as those of his counterpart who's Outwardly Expressive ADD, he would simplify what he saw, slowly turning it into projects and objects once he was in a low-stimulus environment.

Larry exhibited his Alaska-inspired drawings and sculptures—which he made at home after the trip—at arts and crafts fairs. He is the sort of craftsman who sets his work up on easels at the front of his booth, then quietly sits at the back of the booth, partially hidden behind a drape, preferring to talk quietly with one close friend rather than deal with the public. Others may view him as not caring or indifferent. But he's neither. It's just that he feels overwhelmed from too much stimuli: too many people, too many comments, and too many questions. Unless Larry self-protects during the crafts show, he might find that his creativity is diminished afterwards and that he is unable to be creatively productive for a period of time once he gets home.

Ty, in contrast to both Barb and Larry, took Alaska, and everything he confronted, in tow. He may or may not be active like Barb, but his every move is programmed. He's in charge. As someone who's a Highly Structured ADD person, he likes to charge into a situation and take control. But if he can't be in control, he might have great difficulty dealing with the situation.

Ty preplanned his entire trip and forced anyone accompanying him to meet his deadlines and itinerary. Stimulated by a lot of new sights and experiences, Ty spent time every day organizing, categorizing and getting ready for the next events. The more he became stimulated, the more he tried to control everything. He mulled things over in his mind, over and over and over again.

Ty, who also paints, put a heading and page number on the top of every page in his sketchbook. He kept all his pencils and charcoal in one pouch and all his paints in a matching pouch. He could easily locate all his supplies and previous work at a moment's notice.

Ty spent a lot of time getting his materials set up correctly before he began sketching. He eventually sketched and painted, and he was quite brilliant about it. But then he redid the work, improving it and then redid it again. Ty has a hard time feeling satisfied with his work or feeling that a piece is finished. Every new stimulus that came to him would prompt him to redo a piece that was supposedly complete.

Back from Alaska, exhibiting his work for others to view, Ty was still touching it up at the last minute. Gallery directors have a tough time with Ty because he is never satisfied with what he's done and goes around rearranging his pictures while people are coming in for opening night at the gallery.

Barb, Larry, and Ty are all creative artists. Each had a good trip to Alaska and each handled the stimulation they confronted based on their particular form of ADD. None is better nor worse than the others. They are simply each different from one another.

ADD and Sensitivity to Judgment

If you are ADD, you have probably been extremely sensitive to outside judgment for as long as you can remember. In addition, as a creative person, you have opened yourself up to a variety of stimuli. Putting ADD and creativity together, you probably feel very vulnerable when others evaluate your creative products. That evaluation occurs whether or not your work is being formally judged. It really doesn't matter whether your next door neighbor comes in, glances at your production and doesn't say anything, or you've submitted your work to a contest and failed to have it accepted. In both situations, you probably feel a sense of inadequacy about your work and yourself.

Although neither response may have anything to do with the innate quality of your production, your feelings will have been hurt. You are sitting on the inside of your creative, sensitive nature and may well be trying to muster a sense of value about what you do and about yourself, and you feel that your productions represent you.

With heightened sensitivity, you will tend to notice all the reactions, or lack of them, around you. You won't miss the slightest shift of expression or change of tone.

In addition to the many times you feel that you are being judged, there are, of course, those situations in which you really are being openly judged. Teachers, critics, consumers, and competition judges are all commenting on your work in one way or another. As soon as your work is placed on public display, whether it is in a store, a show, or through the media, it becomes fair game for anyone viewing, reading, or listening to critique.

Generally, your own feelings are unimportant to the person who is judging or evaluating your work. Your product is being judged independently of the creative person behind it. Most people just don't think about the fact that this work represents the best effort of the real person who actually created it.

Unfortunately, in many school experiences children are also judged by insensitive teachers who busily mark wrong answers with little thought to the student or to the creative process by which he arrived at his answer. Once they have left the school system they are subjected to bosses, supervisors, creative critics, and others who always have an opinion.

Unfortunately, criticism is usually stated as fact, not as opinion. For example, the critique might read, "The presentation was too long," or "The tempo of the piece was too slow." What needs to be said, instead, is, "The presentation was longer than the evaluator would have liked," or "The evaluator wanted a quicker tempo."

Any of us evaluating and judging another's work must take the responsibility to factor in our own agendas and perceptions—"I wanted to get . . ." rather than "He didn't give me." That takes the sting out of personally challenging and judging a production, while providing grounds for some form of negotiation and improvement later on.

Self-esteem and self-confidence—both of which tend to be problems for people who are ADD in any case—can suffer when work is critiqued carelessly and insensitively. Feelings of inadequacy, even in very talented people, can run rampant.

Even when judgment is positive, it leaves us susceptible to insecurity. That's because we know we have no control over that judgment. If someone has the power to say our work is good, he also has the power to say it is not. We worry about the fact that next time, the pendulum of judgment may swing in the other direction. Our experience has taught us how easily that can happen.

But here's the key: While we cannot control what critics, judges, teachers, or consumers say about our creative products, we do have power over what we think of our work. Ultimately, we must be our own judge. Ask yourself if you met your goals with this creative product. Did you do what you intended to do? Did you meet your own standards of production? Did you create something you like, regardless of what anyone else says? Those are the questions we all need to stay focused on.

I know this is not an easy step to take. That's because most of us feel there is always some outside criteria to meet. But the truth is that no outside criteria can match your own internal one, even though you will often hear differently. Your biggest job is to stand loyally by your own productions, make them the best you can, according to your standards, and then release them into the world knowing that some people will like them and others will not.

While you're learning to develop this sense of positive internal judgment, your reaction to criticism will probably depend on your type of ADD. Remember our three artists who went to Alaska? Let's suppose that each of them enters a juried art exhibit after returning home. Walk with me through the exhibit and let's see how they each react.

Barb, who is Outwardly Expressive, decided to enter her paintings of Alaska in an exhibit. But when she found out that her work had to be judged even to make it into the show, she became angry. "Well, I don't know who these judges think they are," she said. "It doesn't matter whether I get in or not. If I don't get in, it's their loss!"

People who are Outwardly Expressive react to criticism or judgment by mouthing off, criticizing the judges, or making jokes to cover up their sensitivity. Barb will blame everyone but herself for any inadequacies the judges point out in her work. She might even cuss out the judges to her friends. People with this form of ADD aren't really vindictive, but they do tend to blow off steam. When their work receives positive accolades, they can become hyperactive and flamboyant, practically bouncing off the walls.

Although Barb wasn't happy about her work being judged, her pieces did make it into the exhibit. The night of the opening, Barb became hyper, loud, and entertaining. She made it clear to everyone that she didn't want to hear anything negative about her work.

Larry, who is Inwardly Directed, was afraid to enter his Alaska paintings in the exhibit. He knew that if his work didn't make it into the show, he would become very depressed. But when his work was accepted, he wasn't really comfortable being the center of so much attention. Larry kept a low profile. If you had looked for him on opening night, it would have been difficult to find him. Larry was happier being behind the scenes, and he spent most of the night talking to just a few people in the gallery's kitchen.

Someone who's Inwardly Directed would be devastated by negative criticism. He probably wouldn't be willing to show his work again for some time afterward. But he wouldn't say anything openly about the depth of his hurt. In fact, he would probably blame himself, feeling his work was inferior. Being creative, he would probably continue to create, but only in private. The I'm-no-good syndrome frequently takes front row center with people who have this type of ADD.

Ty, who is Highly Structured, spent most of his preshow time worrying. He worked on every detail in each painting to try to get his work absolutely perfect before submitting it for judging. Even so, he kept on worrying. While he was wait-ing, he told his friends that the judges were stupid, and he didn't really care what they thought of his work anyway. Nevertheless, he continued to worry obsessively until he heard from the judges that his work had been accepted.

The opening night of the exhibit, Ty spent most of the evening checking the lights, changing the angle of the shades, fussing with his paintings, and general-ly trying everything he could to completely control the situation. Then late in the evening, he heard someone criticize one of his paintings—and he just blew up. He told the person off, shouting at him in front of everyone that he had no right to pass judgment on someone else's work. Although the crowd became momen-tarily quiet and embarrassed, Ty did not see that as his fault. He was convinced that the problem belonged to the person who had had the nerve to make a neg-ative comment.

People who are Highly Structured can be quite vindictive. It's hard for them to let go of a situation, stop obsessing and move on to something new.

Let's face it. It's never easy for any of us to put ourselves on the line. Personally, I would prefer to have no judges and to just let people display their wares and pro-ductions in a setting that is free from any criticism or judgment. Then let spec-tators gravitate to what they like best—understanding that there is no right or wrong way for work to be, but rather that everyone has different perceptions and will tend to be attracted to what fits them best.

But then, that's my opinion, and I hate criticism! It just hurts too much.

The Goal: A More Positive
Approach to Sensitivity

Almost everyone will tell you that you ought to be willing to listen to criticism and judgment, and that there is a positive, important aspect to it. But I'm not real-ly sure that is true. Every time I try to get myself to agree with the perspective that there is something to be learned from another's criticism, I must weigh it against my opinion of the work and how criticism makes me feel. I want you to at least consider the possibility that you don't have to listen to criticism if you don't want to.

What I do like—and what I've found is helpful to me—is a dialogue with someone knowledgeable, someone who is sensitive to the intent of my work, non-judgmental, and willing to share her ideas that might make the work better. I have had both a writing teacher and two editors who have fit this description. Almost every time we have worked together, I have agreed with their suggestions and been able to accept them with no loss or pain to me.

That's because I don't experience their comments as judgments or evaluations. Rather they seem to be more like partners working with me on my team, with respect for what I'm about. I feel there is a big difference between judgments and critiques and help from someone whose sincere goal is to help me make my work better.

I've shared a bit about how I feel on this subject so that you can contrast your feelings with mine. You might feel very differently than I do. In fact, let's suppose that you do want to have your work critiqued by others. In that case, I'd like to give you some guidelines that may help you sift through what is said and absorb what you want to keep from it.

First, people make their comments based on the way in which they are wired. This includes professionals. That's why one critic will dislike something, and another critic will love it.

For example, I've noticed at national ADD conferences that it is very easy to tell how speakers will be evaluated by those attending the conference, assuming the speaker does a reasonably adequate job.

Speakers who are linear thinkers, follow a tight outline, use slides and talk about what they think or what they have researched get high marks from people who have a lot of Highly Structured ADD. That's because such speakers speak the language of the Highly Structured ADD person and are, in fact, easy for them to understand. There is a mutual language system that is operating in this case, and both speaker and listener feel comfortable with one another.

The same speaker will tend to get lower marks from ADD people who are Outwardly Expressive and people who are creative, analog processors, and like to have a "feelings experience" as listeners. These people might evaluate the outlined, highly structured speaker as boring. But this same group of people will give high marks to a speaker who's Outwardly Expressive and who uses stories, feelings, and empathy as part of her presentation. On the other hand, that type of speaker, as you might guess, will get low marks from listeners who want a clearly defined, orderly, step-by-step presentation about ADD, not a feelings-sense of ADD.

This is one of the reasons that evaluating a presenter doesn't mean much unless you know what the listener responds to and needs. I would rather see extra effort be made to match speakers and participants. Then, rather than evaluations, participant suggestions would guide future presentations.

The second important factor to consider when you are being judged by someone else is the politics that are involved in certain critiques. Most work settings have business and social politics. These are almost always behind the scenes, and the creative person who is concentrating on her work or project may not know that they are operating. But I promise you they are.

This politicking can include interpersonal relationships within the business. Often there are cliques or just friendship circles within businesses, associations, and social groups. If you are a part of such a clique, which may be informal and unstated but present nevertheless, you and your work will tend to be favored.

Critiques also reflect the style that people tend to like or the values that people hold. For example, a group of liberal-minded artists will tend to appeal to liberal-minded viewers. Their work will tend to be included in shows juried by liberal-minded judges. Their work, though of high quality, may be summarily rejected by conservative viewers because of content, rather than artistry. You, as a creative person, need to understand the difference between the two.

What I ask of you is that you don't automatically judge your work or yourself poorly because you get a poor review or lack of attention. It could be that your creativity is ahead of the pack. Or, it could be that your work isn't placed properly in front of an audience or judge who can appreciate what you have to offer.

You must affirm yourself, do the best you can and find people who can appreciate what you do. The ultimate goal is to become self-critical, though not overly so, evaluating your own work by your own standards rather than relying on the judgments of others. Put yourself in the position of being your own ultimate judge.

Know where you are in relation to your own goals. Ask yourself whether you are achieving the way in which you would like to. Do you feel you've made one more step toward the criteria you've set for yourself?

How often do you sense or even know that something is not quite right with a creation of yours, but because you want to be finished with it you don't go back to try to improve it? When you recognize a flaw and you let it slide by, you are setting yourself up to have someone else notice it and comment on it. You need to take responsibility for it and do your best to fix it yourself. You must be true to yourself and have a high level of integrity in relation to your work.

However, although you want to perfect your work as much as possible, I would strongly recommend that you create for the sake of creation first, and for the goal second. Don't create because you're looking for a certain outcome, especially from someone else. Rather let your strong desire to create run the show. Do what you can to make your work the best it can be and then enjoy your creation. Try not to worry about what someone else will say. If your work is really what you want it to be, then criticism cannot hurt you. It can *disappoint* you but not *hurt* you.

When you reach your own goals or achieve what you like with your creative work, you will probably want to share it with others. That's natural. It's kind of like having others "ooh" and "aah" over your baby. It feels very, very good. I understand that it's disappointing when that positive response is not available, but the lack of that response doesn't have to erode your self-esteem or take away from the joy you've found in your work. If someone criticizes a creation that you are satisfied with, you can simply say, "That's interesting. But I see it differently." Then you can choose whether or not to change your work in response to that comment. That way you keep your self-esteem and self-confidence in good shape.

Finally, don't be afraid to ask for what you want. Every creative person will benefit from a close group of friends and colleagues who appreciates his work. Go to them with your completed works and ask for what you want. If it's a work in progress you may want to say, "Any suggestions to make it better?" If you're taking a finished piece that you're satisfied with, you can say, "Tell me how great this is, so I can feel reinforced to take it out into the world at large."

Remember you can't please everyone, so it's good for you to get some real support for work you've finished with which you're satisfied. There's nothing wrong with asking for validation.

YOUR EMOTIONS AND CREATIVITY

Creative people are both very sensitive and very emotional. They experience a broad range of feeling, are aware of what they are experiencing, and know how to use those feelings purposefully as part of their creations. I don't think you can have a creative person who does not work through his emotions.

When creative people express their emotions, they are often misunderstood by their less creative counterparts. The intensity of emotions experienced by a creative person can sometimes be frightening to someone who doesn't share that intensity. The breadth and depth of emotions felt by creative people are sometimes even mistaken for depression, manic-depression, or schizoid personality characteristics.

This is not to say that people who are creative cannot have emotional problems. Of course they can. In fact, many creative and sensitive people carry scars with them from events that would not have hurt a less sensitive person. Also, like anyone else, there are times and situations in which they would benefit from counseling.

As a creative person, it is important for you to become aware of your feelings, learn to manage them, and use them constructively. Counseling can be a positive step in that direction—if you find a counselor who understands the creative personality. Going to counseling does not mean you're crazy. It can help you feel better as you release painful remembrances and learn the coping skills you need to protect yourself.

A teacher or mentor can also sometimes help a sensitive and creative person to learn to manage his emotions. I'm reminded of a man I knew many years ago who was studying harp. I was just beginning my own intense psychotherapy in conjunction with graduate studies in human behavior, and one evening we were discussing how I was learning to deal with my emotions through therapy. He noted that his teacher worked with him a lot on emotions. He was told he wouldn't progress with his mastery of the harp until he dealt with his feelings. He felt that his music teacher—and not a therapist—was the person who could best help him, since the teacher knew what emotional blocks were keeping my friend from improving musically.

Advanced training in many creative fields includes a large emotional component. I've known actresses and actors, musicians and artists who have all had to overcome their own emotional limitations in order to progress in their field. I am certain that, regardless of the area of creative achievement, it is usually a psychological issue—not the lack of talent—that impedes success or advancement. Once that issue is confronted and remedied, creativity can again flow.

Once you've healed past hurts, you need to learn to protect your emotions. I think about it this way: I see my feelings as lying at the center, or core, of myself. Around that core, I've constructed a narrow wall with doorways. The doorknobs are only on one side—so that only I can open and shut the doors. I make the choice of when to open the door and access those emotions. When I determine that it is safe, I open the doors very wide. At other times, I slam them shut emphatically.

You might decide that you need to protect your feelings in other ways, too. For example, one way that I protect myself is by not watching the news. I also don't read newspapers, go to horror movies, or read or see anything with torture or violence. I've learned that being exposed to information about violence affects me deeply and for long periods of time. I do not recover easily, and little is to be gained by continually retraumatizing myself. I know about the abuse and violence in the world and I do what I can. Exposing myself over and over again causes me more pain than I can bear. So I have decided to protect myself from those feelings.

Although I don't hear or read the news, I somehow manage to hear about important local, national, or international events within a day or two. I keep up with trends and watch and observe in my own neighborhood, doing what I can to help out my neighbors. This works for me. This is how I have chosen to protect myself and live, so that I don't totally shut down emotionally.

There's a fine line between learning to protect yourself and walking off from life. Obviously, you don't want to stick your head in the sand and never have any idea of what's going on around you. But the repetitive replay of painful events—

a media habit of recent years—is not constructive for the health of anyone's psyche.

You will know how much to protect yourself. Don't let anyone talk you into situations that hurt you. Don't let anyone shame you or put you down because you choose to protect yourself. You know what's best for yourself.

To maximize self-protection and still stay open to positive stimuli, you have to nurture your emotions from the inside. In order to maintain your creativity, your emotions must be purified, healed, and kept healthy. Wellness training of emotions has to be a part of creative development and care. Self-talk, regular bodywork such as massage, talking with a close friend, meditation, a soothing bath or walk in the woods can all serve to place a balm of soothing nurturance around you.

I would strongly recommend that you find the particular ways that work for you and make them a regular part of your daily life. Don't wait for a crisis. If you do, you'll have to do extra recuperative work before you can begin to build emotional reserves for yourself. You will find that your creativity will actually gain in strength if you nurture yourself regularly. You'll be surprised at the new levels of expression you will reach.

On the other hand, people sometimes use creativity to avoid their emotions or to avoid working on emotional or behavioral issues. For example, people sometimes turn away from a problem in their relationships or business by burying themselves in a creative project. One woman I know started writing a novel rather than face a disintegrating marriage. A man I know, an interior decorator, spent most of every day designing decor, picking fabrics, and seeking exotic accessories, and avoiding his billing and paperwork. Unfortunately, the IRS took a rather dim view of that use of his time, and his business got into serious trouble.

Both the writer and the decorator experienced that wonderful feeling of being taken to another place—a kind of shift in consciousness—that can happen when the creative process is in operation. With their minds away from everyday events, they felt good. Unfortunately, sooner or later, they had to come back to the place they left that didn't feel so good.

Of course, it's fine to use your creativity for R & R or to make you feel better. But you have to know what you're doing. Make a conscious decision to engage in some creative pursuit once you've made plans or arrangements for how to deal with the rest of your life.

Remember to enjoy your creativity and sensitivity, honor it and protect it. Be honest with yourself about it. I know you can do it.

chapter seven

Myths about ADD and Creativity

Y OU AND I will do a lot better in dealing with both ADD and creativity if we learn to recognize the myths that surround them both. These myths are stories, assumptions, or beliefs that have been told and retold year after year, sometimes even passed from generation to generation. Some of the stories are invented, and some were initially based on a real event or situation, but have changed dramatically over time. Unfortunately, many decisions are based on myths. Myths frame what we say and how we act.

For example, consider this myth: If you are thin, you will be happy. Though it's not a myth that is necessarily stated directly anywhere, we tend to see it reflected all around us in commercials and magazine articles, as well as in social conversations, parent-child training, and gossip sessions between friends.

Judy told her mom, "If only I were twenty pounds lighter, I'd have gotten that job, and I wouldn't be so depressed." Convinced that her entire life would be better and she would be happy if only she'd lose that weight, Judy joined an expensive diet program. She did lose that twenty pounds, but she was still not happy. Soon she gained back thirty. It's a common scenario.

Other beliefs in our culture involve money: You will be happy if you have a lot of money. Or how about this one: Doing all your homework will guarantee good grades and later success in life. Or this: If you're honest, life will treat you well.

Many people become bitter when common myths do not produce the results they desire. No wonder! They have believed in something for a long time, and they feel let down or cheated when the results they expect just don't happen.

In this chapter we'll look at some of the common myths associated with ADD and creativity and how they intersect with reality.

COMMON MYTHS ABOUT ADD

Carrie started her sophomore year in high school with strong resolve to make better grades. She eagerly started looking through her books as soon as she got home. She wanted to do well in school, and she was willing to work hard to meet her goal. The second week of school, her science teacher assigned a project that Carrie was very interested in. Carrie jumped right into it, collecting information and planning how she would demonstrate the principles involved and how she would write her paper.

However, after a few days of intense interest, she began to feel discouraged. She had begun to run into problems that she couldn't solve. She couldn't seem to keep her materials organized. Time seemed to be slipping away from her. She found herself focusing intensely on one aspect of the project, then losing track of time and failing to make much overall progress. By the second week of the project she felt totally out of control, unable to dig her way out of the hole she was in. She lost interest in the project.

She went to talk to her teacher about the problems she was having, but her teacher became angry because she thought Carrie just wasn't working hard enough. The teacher said she knew Carrie was smart, and she knew she wanted to make an A on the project. She said she knew Carrie had been excited about the project in the beginning. Why was she just giving up instead of trying harder? Carrie burst into tears.

Several myths associated with ADD are reflected in this story: 1) Carrie's belief that she would be able to organize and carry out the project, because she was interested in the topic and intended to do a good job. 2) Her belief that she could earn a top grade on the project because she wanted to so badly. 3) The teacher's belief that Carrie could succeed if she just tried harder.

Carrie just wanted to be like everyone else who cared about school. She saw that if her peers wanted to make good grades, and they were willing to work hard, they succeeded time after time. But Carrie was running into several major myths about ADD. Which of these ADD myths have touched your life?

Myth 1: *People with ADD would be better off if they would just do things like everyone else.* People with ADD aren't like everyone else. It is a much better idea for them to understand their own particular strengths and weaknesses—and do things in their own way using their strengths to their own advantage—than to try to do things like everyone else.

Myth 2: People with ADD could do it if they just tried hard enough. Unfortunately, even people who are ADD, myself included, have come to believe in this myth very deeply. The result is that we tend to be hard and unforgiving with ourselves. Many ADD adults, especially those generally considered successful, have achieved their accomplishments by overworking, often looking like workaholics. But that's not what's going on. We have to spend those long hours working hard just to keep up.

The biggest problems often lie in organizing and handling the paperwork that results from doing a job. I've even said that maybe I should pull back on the number of business leads I develop, because every lead means having to follow up with paperwork. Some people might interpret that as a fear of success. However, I'm not pulling back because I'm afraid to succeed. I'm pulling back because it is so difficult and overwhelming for me to handle the paperwork. Acquiring and implementing business is a totally different affair than administrating the results and organizing the paper trail that tracks what you've done. I've just discovered, quite by accident, that I was never paid for book sales at a conference three and a half months ago. If someone else hadn't mentioned she'd never been paid, I'd probably have never thought of it again. I don't know how many books were actually sold nor do I have any way to check back. I hope they kept track. That's no way to make a living! Mercy, mercy, spare me from more paperwork!

Myth 3: Anyone who really wants to learn should be able to sit still and pay attention. Unless you, too, have that hyperactive jumping bean inside of you, there is no way to know what it feels like to be expected to sit still when you cannot. It is actually physically painful and really quite impossible. I, like a lot of well-socialized people with ADD, have learned to hold my breath, sit on my hands, or fold my arms across my chest to keep from moving. Although this looks fine from the outside, the result is stiff muscles and discomfort. Ask anyone who is restless and active. We've all felt the same way.

Myth 4: You should finish every project you start. Our culture attaches tremendous value to finishing every project that is started. That's because our culture is more interested in goals and results than in the process of doing things. But for many people with ADD, the process *is* the goal. In other words, for someone with ADD the goal of a particular project might be to learn as much as he can from doing the project. Once he feels he has learned everything he can from the project, he might lose interest. Producing a finished report or display about what he has learned doesn't seem important, and so it doesn't hold his interest.

Obviously, failing to finish work assignments or follow through on commitments can be considered marks of irresponsibility. That's true for everyone, whether you are ADD or not. But most of us also have many projects and interests that could be considered entertainment, or optional. If no one else is counting on you to finish the project, then there's really no necessity to finish if you don't want to.

Just think through the commitments and obligations you've made. Then decide whether or not you can—and whether or not you want to—leave a particular project unfinished. But you also need to realize that, because of ADD issues, even when you decide you want to complete a project, you may become sidetracked and might not always be able to finish in a timely manner.

Myth 5: *You should be responsible for doing all your own work.* In school you are expected to do all your own work without any substantive help from anyone else. Getting help with a paper or help on a test is called cheating. Many of us have those same expectations of ourselves in the workplace. If we are given an assignment, we feel we should be able to do the whole thing ourselves, from beginning to end.

But think about it. How many partnerships have yielded top-notch results, with each partner contributing his or her strength to the whole project? All people have strengths and weaknesses. Why not capitalize on each person's strength, rather than trying to be everything yourself? Fortunately, there is a new trend evolving in the workplace, and wise managers do team up people who have complementary skills. One might be a creative person and the other a good strategist or administrator. That kind of team can work very well and accomplish a lot more than one individual inefficiently trying to do everything alone.

Myth 6: *There are standard and inherently best ways to organize work.* As we've discussed earlier in this book, linear forms of organization are the standard generally accepted as best in this culture. For example, minutes and hours with artificial beginnings and endings are the way people are expected to manage time. Keeping a neat, orderly desk, with all paperwork placed out of sight in files, is considered superior to piles of papers lying about. The ability to break a long-term project down into systematic steps that carry you from a project's beginning straight to its end is considered superior to doing "a little of this" and "a little of that" in no obvious sequence, even if you produce an acceptable product in a timely manner.

But the truth is there are as many ways to accomplish projects as there are people doing them. There is nothing inherently wrong with writing chapter 9 of a book first, followed by chapter 12, chapter 4, and then chapter 1. Neither is there anything wrong with defining a parcel of time by the content of what is being done. Granted, if you are having a conversation that lasts seventy minutes but are trying to fit it into an hour, you've got trouble. But what is so sacred about sixty minutes? Our culture tends to short-change the content of conversations in favor of fitting it into the sixty-minute hour. That's a choice. But it's not necessarily a better or worse choice than letting the content of the conversation define the time slot. Think about it.

When it comes to filing papers and keeping them out of sight, I can tell you that if my papers are out of my sight, I will never think about them again. I keep up with my current work by having stacks of papers, separated into projects, sitting right out where I can find them easily.

As I write this book, I put the chapters in the top slot of a stack tray, where I can readily see them. I have no idea what is in the inner slots because I can't see the papers at a glance. Another book I'm working on is in a brown folder to the left of my answering machine. My travel schedules are stacked on the right side of the desk. Urgent tasks are noted on sticky notes attached to my computer, right in front of my eyes. One note about an urgent task is stuck on the glass door to my house. I can't leave my house without seeing it.

My "filing" system works fine for me. I know where things are, and I can get to them in a timely manner. If I put active work in folders and file them, I can never remember how I labeled them or where to find them. When I finish a project, I get great joy from filing them out of sight. It's a celebration.

Myth 7: People who are ADD shouldn't be so sensitive. And clouds shouldn't rain. You already know my opinion on this one. We are as sensitive as we are—and that's that!

Myth 8: People who are ADD should be able to control their emotions and be less re-active. Given the level of sensitivity most of us are endowed with naturally, we react exactly to the degree that makes sense. Just because we live in a culture in which the majority believes emotional inhibition is better than expression doesn't mean there is anything wrong with being emotionally expressive. The trick, of course, is to be able to decide when to express and when to curtail those emotions. But given the sensitivity of people who are ADD, it's not surprising that it takes a number of years to learn those skills of inhibition. Those skills do come in time. But it's a myth to think that a sensitive person can just turn emotions on and off.

Myth 9: It's always best to reach your goal by the shortest route. Direct progress to the goal, though efficient, may not provide much quality to life. Neither does it allow room for creativity to blossom. Taking a leisurely, circuitous route to a goal is different than taking the shortest route—but not necessarily less valuable. The trick is to decide what kind of trip you want to take, and then take it. Ask yourself some questions. Do you have time to look at the scenery? Do you have time to develop options and be creative? Do you have a time crunch that is important to honor?

Obviously, to use an extreme example, if a person in an emergency room is dying because of restricted breathing you want to get him breathing as soon as possible, using the shortest, straightest way to make that happen. But most situations are not that clear cut. Suppose, for example, that a person wants to set up a physical training program. He may want to try out a number of different types of training techniques, cross-training options, and alternative activities to see what he likes best and what is effective for his particular body. There's no rush, and taking the time in the long run for trial and error and exploratory activities will yield the results that fit the individual best, at least for the time being.

Myth 10: People with ADD attributes are not as smart, or as capable of learning, as their non-ADD peers. Nothing could be farther from the truth than this myth. Not only are people who are ADD as smart as their non-ADD peers, but those who manage to stay out of big trouble are probably smarter. It's just that ADD people are not necessarily smart at the same things as non-ADD people.

Our culture uses the word "intelligence" to mean mostly verbal and mathematical intelligence. But there are many other kinds of intelligence. Even verbal and mathematical intelligence are often measured in a non-ADD way.

For example, take a child's ability to do math in his head. Many ADD children can do this quite successfully. But they get into trouble when they must commit their figuring to paper. An ADD child makes "careless" mistakes because his mind wanders, and he loses concentration between arriving at the answer and writing it down. On the paper, he might mark the wrong answer. All that really proves is that the child has problems doing paperwork—which is no surprise in relation to ADD. Unfortunately, our culture usually takes that incorrect answer as a superficial measure of the child's intelligence.

The instructional methods used in most schools do not favor people with Outwardly Expressed or Inwardly Directed ADD. But put them in a hands-on, apprenticeship model of learning, and they will often learn rapidly. Students with Highly Structured ADD tend to hyperfocus, and they often do quite well with the current mode of education.

Myth 11: People who are ADD are deficient or disordered. People who are ADD are often labeled deficient or disordered because the person giving out those labels is a very highly focused linear thinker. He or she probably did well in school, liked paperwork, and was successful later on the job. He or she assumed that anyone who didn't have those characteristics was deficient.

I have no problem being called deficient in relation to managing paperwork and the organization of administrative details—I know and acknowledge that that is not my forte. But I do object to being called deficient or disordered as a general description of my character, as if I were deficient in all kinds of ways. In reality, I am very efficient at organizing my inner feelings, keeping track of the most minute details of those feelings, remembering the subtlety of the tones of colors that may go into an artistic work or the musical tones that I put together to replicate my inner feelings when I am setting them to music.

Attention *Deficit Disorder* is a total misnomer, and it needs to be changed.

Myth 12. It takes an exceptional amount of work to teach someone who is ADD. Though being taught *about* things—through the traditional system of reading and lectures—is difficult for a lot of ADD people, being trained to learn mental and physical skills is not. We are trainable, even if we are not readily educable *about* things. What I mean by this is that training (a process of repeating an activity or process in practical ways until it is learned) is a better method of teaching people who are ADD than teaching in the abstract or out of context.

So, if you want to teach the principles of sociology to a student with ADD, provide the student with stories and examples of the principle at work, rather than telling about the principle or having the student read about it. Show the principle in operation and the ADD student will tend to understand it and retain it readily.

Training also means repeatedly walking a person through the steps needed to learn something, especially when it comes to skills that are difficult for people with ADD to master, such as keeping track of gas mileage or balancing a checkbook. It may take repeated trials to instill the habit. But once the habit is learned, it tends to stick. How different from studying for a test in which a student performs well, only to lose the information, or ability to use the information, shortly after the test.

Myth 13. Most people who are ADD need medication to function well and live up to their potential. I'm not against using medication at all. In fact I have seen it work miracles for people who have never been able to think one thought at a time, sit still for ten seconds or maintain attention on a task for even a short time. But not everyone with ADD automatically wants or needs medication.

The decision about whether or not to use medication depends on many factors. If a student is required to sit still at a school desk and pass tests on the content of lectures, medication might be helpful. But medicating a stand-up comic who is taking in information from his audience and instantly transforming it into jokes and comedy routines is ludicrous.

Remember that ADD has as many positive aspects as negative. Whether or not any individual needs medication depends upon what the person is trying to accomplish. One thing is for certain, though. If you take medication only—without associated training to improve your skills—you will not be doing yourself justice. Never just take medication and expect that it will solve all your problems like a magic bullet.

Anyone who is ADD requires training and education to understand and build behavioral and emotional skills to cope in a non-ADD culture. You can learn to better control your attention, impulsivity, and emotions. You can learn the organizational skills you need to manage time, details, and paperwork more efficiently. You can learn to break long-term projects into small, manageable segments. If you can study these skills in a training program with others who are ADD, then you can also benefit emotionally from the camaraderie. You *can* reach your potential. But medication will never be the entire answer.

Myth 14: People with ADD attributes need treatment for their problem. ADD is not a disorder requiring treatment. But because people who are ADD live in a world that does not at this time favor their characteristics, professionals often think treatment is necessary to correct what is "wrong." Instead, I would suggest that you seek training and education to learn specific skills that will help you fit into the existing culture. The goal is not to change you to become something different from who you are. You are not meant to be a non-ADD, linear person. You can stay basically as you are and honor and respect your unique strengths, but add a few skills that will help you do better as you cope with a non-ADD culture in your day-to-day living.

The "problems" associated with ADD are often secondary problems that occur from living in a world that does not accept or value the ADD style. People who are wired in an ADD way are not given the opportunity to learn coping strategies for use in a non-ADD world—the strategies that are taught are usually taught in a non-ADD way. They are also not taught to develop their innate ADD skills. As a result, they neither adapt to the non-ADD world in which we live nor learn to utilize their innate skills effectively.

The result is a group of secondary problems for ADD people that include depression, low self-esteem, chemical abuse and other self-medicating behaviors, feelings of inadequacy, unmanaged tempers, and underachievement. Many people who are ADD have also suffered traumas from personal abuse and from being raised by parents equally frustated because of their lack of information about ADD. These parents have developed few, if any, coping skills.

Counseling, though useful for the treatment of emotional and behavior disabilities, is not helpful for the ADD attributes. Save counseling for the secondary problems associated with ADD. But even then the counselor must understand the effects of ADD brain wiring and structure the counseling appropriately. Adaptations must also be made to recovery programs and counseling techniques of all kinds if they are to be effective with people who are ADD. A lot of time and money has been wasted because counselors did not adjust for ADD with their clients.

Remember, counseling does not "fix" ADD nor does it teach people with ADD how to cope in a linear world. Training and education can teach those needed skills.

Myth 15: People who are ADD get off track—and they need to do something about that. When we say someone has gotten off track, what we usually mean is that the person didn't take the most direct route from point A to point B. But as we discussed in chapter 4, the most direct route is not always the best route. It just depends on what your goals are. You can decide how you want to live your life and the goals you want to strive for. And then you can proceed on any route you'd like. The path you choose doesn't necessarily need to be a clear and straight path just to make others happy. You can do what's best for you.

COMMON MYTHS ABOUT CREATIVITY

Jacob, a twenty-four-year-old mechanic, toured the country working on race cars. Drivers trusted him because he had a special talent—Jacob could fix absolutely anything. Working quickly under pressure never bothered him. In fact, Jacob seemed to thrive on those it-just-can't-be-done situations. He always got it done—on time. Then when the pressure was off, he would develop a better part or a better way to wire a car to avoid that problem in the future. Jacob was incredibly creative. After hours he enjoyed the company of the people he worked with, several of whom were also very creative.

Though he didn't make enough money to really save any, he did earn enough to support himself. Every few weeks, he would decide to see a new part of the country, ask for references—he always got good references—and take off on his next adventure. He was happy.

But every time he spoke with his parents, they wanted to know when he was going to settle down and get a "real" job. They thought he was just fooling around. When he explained that he loved the challenge and the creativity of his work, his parents replied that it wasn't "real" work. "Real" work to them meant wearing a suit and working in an office building.

Jacob's parents had bought into the myth that a real job involves stability, not creativity. That's just one of the myths surrounding creativity. Let's look at some of the others.

Myth 1: Creativity has little value in the work-a-day world. It's just an extra. With the exception of a very obvious talent, most creative interests and activities are thought of as extracurricular—something you do if you have time after your "real" work is done. But the truth is that creative interests can be put to work to earn an adequate, and often very good, income, and they can provide a person with a very happy life.

If you are a creative thinker and live a creative lifestyle, you can bring your creative talents to any job. You can make a contribution in the workplace, and even extend that contribution into the world.

Everything is founded on creativity: the beginning of a new business, the construction of a new design, the development of any new idea. Without creativity, nothing would be accomplished. There would be no zest, no new beginnings, and no change. Creativity is not just an extra. It rests at the very heart of all we know and have.

Myth 2: Creative people will not be able to make a good living. Some creative people hit it big. Most don't. But even when creative artisans make less money than their corporate counterparts, they often come out just as well off in the long run — after you've factored in net gain in joy of living. I'm serious. I'm not just trying to be a Pollyanna here.

It's difficult to calculate how much financial security a person has and what it means. A person can exhibit all of the outward signs of success: a beautiful home, new car, lots of clothes. But that person might be up to his ears in debt and very unhappy. On the other hand, someone who earns less might be living within his means and have a full life of companionship and the joy of being creative — even if that someone's parents don't think he has a real job.

Deciding what a good living is involves making judgments. Does it mean that your income is just enough to pay your rent or mortgage? Does it mean you can afford extracurricular lessons for your kids or save money for their college educations? Or is it the ability to take costly vacations to foreign lands?

Being creative can also mean being financially creative in obtaining what you want. Making trades for services with others, networking to obtain what you want, and figuring out ways to get what you want while someone else agrees to pay the bills may be the rule rather than the exception with creative people.

Myth 3: Creative people are troublemakers because they don't follow the rules or stay within the limits set by society. Our culture tends to identify someone as a troublemaker if he fails to stay within the rules or standards set by others, or just generally do things differently from the norm. But I see things another way. If someone's behavior is outside the narrow bounds of society but within the limits of the law, that person is not necessarily causing trouble. Young people particularly come to mind in this case. It is the nature of adolescence to challenge the status quo, but teens who do things differently are often labeled as troublemakers. If you stop and think about it, what's really so awful about dressing in a funky way or not wanting to abide by stuffy, stifling rules that prohibit males from wearing long hair or an earring on the job? Does it really matter whether or not you have a mustache? Isn't it more important that you bring in business and relate well to the customers?

Graffiti on public buildings is another good example. In communities where specific areas have been set aside for public expression, people are generally more than willing to restrict their artistry to those areas. The quality of the artistic creations also improves. Often young people truly have little to do to amuse themselves and few ways to express their creativity. So, being creative, they make things up to amuse themselves. The form it takes may be inappropriate. But if you read the intent of the missteps, you will find a creative urge for activity that can be readily channeled.

Myth 4: The creative way of doing things is not efficient. If you were to undertake a time-and-motion study of creative people, you would probably discover that they experiment with many different ways of doing things in their journey to a goal. The goal, after all, is to create something new, not to efficiently replicate something that has already been created. That's what creativity is all about! Without experimentation, side-road excursions, and trial and error, there would be no creativity. In creativity it's the process and, to some extent, the product that's important. Efficiency is not the goal of creativity.

Myth 5: You can't be creative and responsible at the same time. The key to understanding the origin of this myth is to understand the term "responsible." What seems responsible to one person might be irresponsible to another. One person might consider it a responsible act to keep track of every gas purchase, miles driven, and tax paid on gasoline. Someone else might see that same act as an irresponsible waste of time.

For example, consider Carolyn. When Carolyn was put in charge of organizing a community project, she considered ways to excite the participants about improving their lot in life. She created a new approach to reaching the participants and created new programs. A large portion of the community became involved in the project, and Carolyn considered it a success.

But her boss was not happy with her work. He said she spent too much time being creative and not enough time collecting statistics—statistics that he could put in his report to the project's underwriting agency. He told Carolyn she needed to be more responsible.

Although Carolyn was not at all interested in collecting numbers, she recognized that her boss had not communicated his needs clearly to her. Her boss, not a particularly creative man, assumed Carolyn understood that the main goal of the program was the accumulation of data. Carolyn assumed that the main goal of the program was taking care of people.

It wasn't that Carolyn was irresponsible. It was that her values were different from her boss's and didn't fit his needs and agenda.

Myth 6: Creative people don't have their feet on the ground. Dreaming, visioning, and experimenting often make a person seem like he is "out to lunch." But it's really just another way of living.

Generally, having your feet on the ground means something very specific to those who use that phrase. It means going about what you're doing in a direct, sequential manner and working toward a goal without taking side trips to investigate things of interest.

For example, when Hans, who was working in a chemistry lab to develop better bonding techniques, started working instead on a whole new chemical process, he was told that he needed to get practical. "Get your feet back on the ground," his boss said. After all, the lab needed the money from the original job for business purposes. But Hans realized that the new process he was exploring could potentially bring in even more money to the lab. He had already asked his lab partner to continue the original job so that he could explore the new possibilities.

Granted, there are some creative people who do get off track and don't live in a practical way, according to commonly held standards and values. But if they manage to live in a self-sufficient manner, not dependent on others, there is really no need to be judgmental about their choices.

Myth 7: The creative way of thinking is just not as good as the no- nonsense, linear way of doing things. As we've discussed previously, thinking in a linear, sequential, empirical way is generally considered to be superior in our culture. Creative, analog thinking is appreciated when it yields superior creations. But when applied to everyday learning, especially in academic settings that are based on empiricism and research-oriented results, creative thinking is often considered inferior. The workplace also tends to reflect the thinking of the academic world, and linear thinking is usually considered superior to creative analog thinking.

But it's really all just a matter of values, so think about the situation you find yourself in and decide which form of thinking works best for you in that setting and which manner of thinking you prefer. Then go for it!

Myth 8: Creativity has no structure or form; the creative process has little structure or form. Creativity does have a structure—it's just a different structure than that of other processes. The apparent haphazardness that is often displayed in the creative process reflects the different ways in which thinking happens. The criteria used by a creative person for judging progress, goals, and accomplishments are not always readily apparent to the outside observer. If you ask the creative person why he does what he does in a certain order, he'll probably be able to tell you—and it will make sense. But creative people are not likely to offer such an explanation, because it's not important to them.

Myth 9: If children are creative, then anyone can be creative—so it's no big deal. Besides, that means being creative is childlike. Yes, children are naturally creative. Most of us were creative as children. It's the socialization and learning processes that steer us in other directions, away from continuing to exercise our creativity. Growing up is associated with doing things in the culturally accepted way. That means leaving creativity behind in childhood or, at least, the creative way of doing things, and becoming socialized and efficient.

Being able to display specific creative talents may be acceptable for adults in our culture, but living a creative lifestyle is not, because it involves trial and error and experimentation. "Learn to get it right," "Stop messing around," "Hurry up," are all phrases that are leveled at growing children. With such judgments coming at them, is it any wonder that children learn to leave their creative ways behind?

Yes, children can be creative. But that doesn't lessen the value of creativity — unless you believe that children have less value as people than adults do.

Myth 10: You can't really be creative unless you have a special talent. As we've discussed previously, there are two aspects to creativity. One is the emergence of a creative or special talent. The other is living a creative lifestyle in which you take a creative approach to everything you do. Creativity in this sense is a part of the fabric of your entire life.

Many people who are generally creative do not have a special talent that is highly developed. But they might do many things well and enjoy creative problem solving. Although they might not be known for one specific talent or skill, they are, nevertheless, highly creative.

Myths Affecting Both ADD and Creativity

ADD and creativity are not the same thing. In some ways they are completely separate issues. But they do share some striking similarities. If you are ADD, our culture holds many myths concerning your talents and behaviors that are similar to the myths about creativity. If you are creative, you will be sensitive to what people who are ADD go through because you will have experienced many of the same blocks and beliefs that have made things difficult for them.

Whether you are ADD or creative you have been wounded time after time by common misunderstandings about the ways in which you function, how you go about doing what you do, and even about your character and goals in life.

But, in reality, you are just a person who is doing the best you can, just like everyone else. Your intent always was, is, and always will be to do the best you can. And, like everyone else, you can only do things in the way that fits you.

You didn't intend to cause trouble, be inferior, or not fit into the status quo — at least, not until fitting in proved to be impossible. Then, recognizing your inability to fit in comfortably, you may have opted to go as far away from the status quo as possible.

I recall many years ago when I was working in a school in West Los Angeles. By fourth grade, most kids in the school were considered to be against "the system." In an attempt to understand that situation, I spoke to a colleague who was very familiar with the area. He told me something I've never forgotten. He said,

"All kids start out wanting to be 'good' so they can be accepted. But if that becomes impossible because of circumstances beyond their control, they would rather be really 'bad' than in the middle. In the middle means that you're no one and that feels awful. At least when you're 'bad,' you're someone." How true! I understood.

People who are different, whether it's because of ADD or their creative nature or both, will eventually find out that they can't "get it right" in this very linear society. So they not only quit trying to do things in acceptable ways but will often become atrociously different. Underneath, let's not forget that each of us wants to be accepted. Yet we must be who we are. Our identity can't be changed or taken away. And this is, by the way, one of the main reasons why levels of depression are so high in our society: We have a rigid standard of acceptance with a low level of tolerance for differences.

Not being able to "get it right" brings us to the most important underlying myth about ADD and creativity:

ADD AND CREATIVITY ARE LESSER WAYS OF BEING.

Think about what that means. Do you feel that society looks at you as being inferior to the standard of the culture? Probably so. If you are ADD or creative, society tends to look down on you and your way of doing things as being less valuable than the acceptable, linear standard. Devaluation of your way of being and that lack of understanding can take its toll. Then you realize how important it is for others to at least make an effort to understand you and perceive your value.

Part of what happens is that in the early years of education, creativity and/or the ADD way of learning is treated as inferior. From that experience we learn that our way of *being* is inferior, though no one intended to teach us that. When we grow up, we continue to carry this belief with us. Even though there will be other adults who do respect our way of doing things or think we are acceptable just the way we are, we continue to assume that we are inferior, because that is what we learned early on.

If your family honors creativity, or if some of your family members can serve as creative models, you will develop a more solid foundation upon which to build. But even if your family doesn't buy into the myth of inferiority, you will still be assaulted by different beliefs when you go out into the world.

Some families, not knowing any better, simply fail to recognize and encourage their children's differences. Those children are hurt by default. Some families actively encourage their children to be like everyone else and do things the "right" way.

But regardless of the circumstances in which you were raised, if you are ADD and creative you will have to reconcile your relationship to the majority culture at some time in your life. Right now can be just the time to do it. The alternative is to buy into the myth that you are inferior. If you do that, you will have lost a precious part of you. You'll feel nothing but bad about the wonderful way that you are.

Buying into the myth ourselves is one of the most serious problems that those of us who are ADD and creative have. After all, what we believe about ourselves is key to making us happy. If we don't feel we are up to par, then we'll never feel very good about ourselves.

If you truly think you *should* be able to sit still for an hour doing paperwork, then you will feel bad every time you fail to do that. If you truly think you *should* be content with a boring job when you dream to be able to do creative work, then you will feel guilty about your desire and inadequate about your abilities.

Buying into the myth of inferiority creates emotional problems galore. Depression surfaces quickly, often accompanied by feelings of guilt. Anxiety, panic attacks, and compulsive behavior may also be present. Then there are the mood swings. When we are trying to do what doesn't fit us properly, we are likely to feel depressed. When we occasionally are able to do something that fits us, our mood may soar so high that others, not understanding what is happening, will think we've become manic.

In addition to problems with our feelings, our behavior may suffer. Impulsivity, temper problems, anger outbursts, and oppositional behavior can result if people buy into that myth of inferiority. And many people who buy into that myth start lying. That's because they believe they are inferior and want to cover up so others won't see that.

Impulsivity is one of the most obvious behavioral issues for ADD or creative people who feel inferior to the general culture. If, for example, you see a little window of opportunity to do something creative, you may impulsively try to dart through to catch that opportunity that you feared you might not have. Suppose you are in a job that is boring and you want to be doing something creative. If someone comes along who seems to recognize your ability and says he will support you in business, you might just quit your job on the spot and begin to produce your creative work without doing the research that really is necessary before you start a new business.

Many times people make promises or *seem* to understand what a creative person is about, but they don't have the skill to follow through to bring the creative work to market so that both of you can make a living. The next thing you know, your new-found business partner has not produced the market you need, left you in the lurch, and you are without a job to pay your rent. That's a tough situation.

You will be blamed for acting impulsively. In fact, you will probably blame yourself as you listen to others who try to advise you against such moves in the future.

What you should realize from that type of experience is that the creative drive is very strong and seeking expression. Add ADD to this scenario and you have double trouble lying in wait for you. Yes, you need to get your impulsivity under control, but I can promise you that it may take years for you to stop chasing rainbows. You will only stop when you finally realize that you must take your time and do some research rather than automatically believing what others say and jumping into inviting-looking situations without thinking. You will have learned by having been burned.

All in all, the feelings and behaviors associated with buying into the myth of inferiority do not make a pretty picture. They are well worth avoiding. So I want you to step back and look at what you believe about yourself. Go over the myths listed earlier in this chapter about ADD and creativity. Check the ones that fit you.

Are you willing to think about these myths and label them inaccurate?

I believe they are all wrong and do not fit any of us. I am basing that decision on years of experience working with people who are ADD and creative, and the fact that I know the myths are wrong for me—and wrong for you. But you must come to your own decision for yourself. Then you can escape from the self-judgment, self-evaluation and the self-defeating mode that comes when you believe wholeheartedly in something that is inaccurate about you.

CHANGING YOUR MYTHS

I have spent thousands of hours listening to people's stories and helping them look at their belief systems. I've been able to help many people change their beliefs so that they become self-supporting and self-appreciative. That is not to say that it is my business to *make* anyone change—not you or anyone else. But when the mirror is held up so that you can see who you really are, you will see the wonderful person you are meant to be—not a misshapen reflection of what someone else thinks you *should* be.

I want to give you a process that you can use to change any belief that *you choose*. It is a process that engages your thinking mind as well as your feelings. It allows you to rework any belief that you accepted long ago, when you couldn't think about what you were learning, and you simply absorbed beliefs without thinking. This is a five-step process, and by the end of the fifth step, you will be able to make a *conscious* decision to either change what you've believed and create a new belief, or leave the old one the way it was.

If you choose to leave the old idea intact, then that belief is no longer a myth.

It is a belief that you have truly made your own through a conscious effort. In that case you will believe deeply in that concept and, consequently, you won't feel sad, depressed, anxious, or resentful because you are trying to do something that you think you *should* do.

As an example, let's use a myth that causes trouble for both creative and ADD people: *Your way of doing things is not the best way.*

To begin, ask yourself the following questions:

1. *From whom did I learn my belief in the first place? Who or what situations taught me that my way of doing things was not the best way?*

After you've asked yourself the question, sit still and see what comes to mind. You might get a mental picture or hear some dialogue from years earlier. Whatever comes to mind will tend to help you answer this question. Maybe someone in your family believed her own way of doing things wasn't right and went around saying, "I never do anything the right way." If that were the case, you would have learned by watching a model.

2. *Did I learn my belief because I was afraid not to believe that way or because I wanted someone's approval?*

Again notice what comes to mind. Were you afraid that you'd be punished or scolded for the way you did things? Maybe you were embarrassed or overheard others talking about you. You might have received a disapproving look from one of your parents.

On the other hand you may have been praised every time you did something in a way that *wasn't* natural for you. Though the people around you didn't necessarily show disapproval of your natural ways, you learned that the way you would be accepted was by doing it "right."

In the first situation you learned by fear. In the second, by your need for approval. You will find that it is easier for you to change your myth now if you were only seeking approval than if you were also afraid. You will need to help protect the child within you if you were raised with fear.

3. *What new information do I have to consider that may change my original viewpoint?*

You've been doing a lot of reading in this book about the nature of ADD and the nature of the creative person. That may be new information for you. Think about what you've learned about basic neurobiochemical wiring—that we are the way we are because that is how we are put together. Remember, also, how many of the standards by which we are judged have been set by people who are wired differently and simply haven't understood the ADD and creative styles.

4. What are some of the side effects or costs of your old belief?

Ask yourself whether or not you have been suffering from low self-esteem, guilt, resentment, depression, physical symptoms such as headaches and other pains, or behavioral difficulties such as eating or drinking too much. Any of these could be the side effects or costs of your old belief.

5. What new feelings do you have about your old belief?

Feel your feelings, not what you *think* but what you *feel*. Perhaps you begin to feel a sense that your way can be just as good as, though different from, the way other people do things. Maybe you feel sadness for having lived so long trying to be someone different from who you really are.

Now that you have answered those five questions for yourself, it's time to consider your alternatives. You can actively decide—and this is where the thinking process comes in—whether or not you want to keep the belief that you really *should* be like other people and that there is something wrong with the way you do things. Or you can decide that you want to set the old myth aside and form a new belief—one that says that your natural way of doing things is just fine.

If you choose to continue to believe in the original myth, and you still feel inadequate and bad, I would suggest that you are still trying to do something that doesn't fit you and you may need to continue to work, perhaps through counseling, on finding a fit that can work better for you.

If you choose to change the old myth to one that says something like, "*My way of doing things is just fine,*" then I ask you to do a little ritual to complete the transaction at hand. Consider the old you who lived with the myth. Acknowledge empathetically that you really tried hard to live by that belief and that a lot of misunderstanding surrounded you. Forgive the old you for not being able to live up to the myth and explain to the old you that the reason was because it didn't fit you.

Next say good-bye to the old myth. Visualize the old you who believed it and say "thank you" to that part of you and release that part with a hug. Next reach out in your imagination to the present you and offer the new belief. Say, "Your way of doing things is just fine." As you visualize yourself currently, extend a hand

and welcome the new way of looking at the world. Make a commitment to live by the new belief that "I'm okay just the way I am."

Now the belief fits you and your present situation. No more myths. You are free to be who you were always meant to be.

Remember you can use this five-step process to change any myths or beliefs that you automatically held without thinking. By going through the steps, you marry your feelings with your thinking in a context that fits you. Keep your eyes open for myths that need this type of challenge.

You can now draw the conclusion that you are an ADD/creative person who is exactly the way you were always meant to be. You can affirm the way you are. And you'll find that as you affirm yourself and your way of doing things, others will, too.

You will have overcome the myths that trapped you so that you can build a new paradigm in which to exist. And be sure to make that new paradigm self-affirming and joyous.

chaptereight

Reinstating Creativity

ELEN SPENT thirty-five years working as a counselor. Thanks to her innate creativity, she gained considerable success designing programs that really helped young students who were having trouble staying in school. She was also creative in her ability to talk with and counsel students, and each of her relationships with the students was unique. Her students benefited greatly from Helen's talents and never forgot that she made such a difference in their lives.

However, Helen did not experience the joy her students felt. She didn't feel like she was being creative. She subtly mourned being out of touch with her own creativity.

It's not that she didn't appreciate what she did for her students—it's just that she didn't think of it as being creative. Because of this, she felt like something very important was missing from her life. As a child, Helen had dreamed of being an artist. She painted the visions in her mind on paper. More than anything, Helen wanted to be creative.

But it wasn't until after she retired from her professional job that she turned her attention back to the visions and dreams of her youth. It's interesting that, as soon as she did, she also became free of depression for the first time in years. Her level of anxiety diminished, too.

Though there may be many reasons for these emotional changes, I'm certain that part of the issue has to do with the fact that Helen had felt out of touch with her creativity—a natural, important part of her identity. When she corrected that situation, she felt wonderful.

Helen positively glows these days when she's painting. Her work is beautiful and so is her smile. You should see her when she's teaching young children about art! Helping them to stay connected to the creative parts of themselves seems to be helping Helen heal, too.

THE PROCESSES AT WORK IN RECLAIMING YOUR CREATIVITY

The process of reconnecting to creativity happens in several typical ways. But there is always one common element: a trigger. Something happens in your life and it serves as a trigger for you to realize that you want to and can get back to your creativity and start really using it again.

One typical trigger, like Helen's, is age or stage in life. Retirement obviously allows for time to engage in creative work. It may allow you to turn to creativity now that you no longer need to be a "serious adult" engaging in practical matters. This particular trigger is very much influenced by the cultural belief that you can't make a living being creative. Now, retired, you have permission to spend your time being creative.

Aging also brings a change in values for most people. Money may become less important than doing what you love to do. Being the person you truly feel you are inside may become more important than mechanically doing what you feel you *should* do. That may open the door for you to enjoy your creativity.

Another common trigger also causes a change in values. If you suffer an illness or threat to your life, you may find a strong feeling emerging that says, "I must do what is important to me in the time I have left." It really doesn't matter how much time that is. What matters is the intensity with which you desire to be who you naturally feel you are—to express the *real* you.

Maybe you have recently gained control over your own mental health or are in recovery from some form of substance abuse, and seeing the world more clearly. At times like these your values change, and your motivations become more apparent to you. By being free of active substance abuse or addictive behavior, you come to more truly know who you are and what you want, what's important to you in the bigger scheme of things. Hurrah for you!

Maybe your trigger is the fact that your children are beginning school. That change frees up several hours during the day. Maybe your grown children are leaving home for college or work. Maybe your spouse got a raise that gives you the opportunity to quit work. Maybe you inherit family money that makes you feel as if you can spend time in a way that pleases you. Any of these types of lifestyle changes would allow you to do something you *really* want to do.

In fact, anything that causes a major change in your life can also be a catalyst for deciding to reclaim lost creativity. And I do mean *deciding*. Regardless of the catalyst, ultimately you must decide to reach out—or reach within yourself—to lay claim to what has always been your right, your creativity.

By listening to your inner feelings, you will be guided to know what you are made of. If you are sad because you are not *feeling* creative or feel separated from your creativity, then I promise you that means you are creative and your feelings are trying to let you know how much you yearn to be connected to that part of you.

Anything that causes you to listen to your inner feelings can bring you to this point: recovery programs, counseling or psychotherapy, meditation and spiritual growth, or wellness activities.

But you must decide to listen to your inner feelings. Listening to what's in your heart can then become a catalyst for reclaiming your lost creativity. My advice would be to listen carefully. Notice what makes you happy. Notice what makes you feel thrilled and how you feel when you tingle inside with excitement and anticipation.

The next step is giving yourself permission to be creative. To give yourself that permission, you have to examine your old belief systems and ask yourself how you lost your creativity in the first place. You have to reconnect with that part of you that was told you *shouldn't* be creative. You may wish to have an inner dialogue with the part of you that was trained to reject your creativity. That may be a dialogue with a child part of you or a dialogue with the young adult part of you who was entering "the serious world of adulthood."

If you are a visual person you may want to visualize that part of you that was trained to reject your creativity. Or you may wish to role play, write a poem, a script or story about that part. Maybe, like Helen, you want to work out your permission by teaching children about the area of creativity in which you are interested.

Next, turn to the person you're addressing within yourself and say, "It's okay. I, the adult, am going to take over now. I choose to give you, the creative part of me, permission to be expressive." And then rejoice in your new connection. Don't be surprised if you shed a tear or get a lump in your throat. That's what happens when we come in contact with an old loved one after a time of separation.

Exercises for Reclaiming Your Lost Creativity

As we discussed in chapter 3, your natural creativity is based on the natural unfolding of the Core Components of Human Nature—trust, identity, competence, power, and self-control. Now that you have identified the fact that you do want to reclaim your lost creativity, you can go through the stages that helped you grow when you were young—when your creativity was ready to naturally unfold. By doing this, you will reconstruct the pathway that would have provided you with a connection to your creativity as a young child. This time, as an adult, you will not lose touch with your creativity along the way.

You'll find exercises below that coincide with the development of each core component. You may want to spend more time with resuscitating one component than another because it may be that one was not well developed when you were young or it became damaged later. For example, maybe you were so highly socialized as a child that you engaged in the activities that your parents wanted rather than doing what *you* wanted to do, so your identity was compromised. But you did have lots of opportunities to develop feelings of competence about what you did. In a case like that, for example, you might want to spend more time working on identity development than working on your sense of competence.

These exercises are something you can do by yourself for yourself. Of course, you can share what you are doing with others, but you don't need to do that for the exercises to be effective. It doesn't take special training or tutoring to accomplish them. In the process you will gain the specific guidance you need to reawaken your creativity. Do one exercise at a time. Don't rush. Check the ones you have completed.

Trust

In this situation when I say "trust," I mean trusting that your needs will be met. When dealing with that sense of trust, you must, as an adult, learn to ask for what you want from others. As a child you may have cried to get what you want. Now, that would not be very well received—though many adults still do it. Instead, simply learn to ask.

> **EXERCISE 1.** This week, go to someone you know who tends to be kind or generous and ask that person to help you. Don't apologize for asking or take a lot of time saying why you need the help. Just ask for the help you need simply and in a straightforward manner. You might want to try asking someone to switch lunch periods with you, or help you take your car in for an oil change. Keep your request simple. If you are turned down, ask a sec-

ond person, and remember, we are all sometimes turned down for what we need, but that doesn't mean we can't trust someone else.

When you receive what you've asked for, say "Thank you." Then take a deep breath and tell yourself, "I asked and I received. This time I got something I needed. This is a building block for learning to trust."

EXERCISE 2. Learning to trust yourself is important, too. If, in taking a new job, you fear you won't be accepted or liked by the other employees, you are likely to hear a voice in your mind saying, "No one will like me. I'll have to eat lunch all alone." Recognize that you learned those beliefs either from past experience or from something you were taught as a child.

Change the program now. Demand that you speak well and kindly of yourself, whether you believe what you say or not. Say, "I will succeed. I am likable." Corny? Maybe. Essential for positive outcomes? Totally. Just do it. After all, what do you have to lose except pain and failure? Can you stand that? You bet.

EXERCISE 3. Learn to gain nurturance for yourself and your creativity. Seek out a mentor or a small group that is supportive of what you are doing. Be cautious to select people who are gentle, positive, and flexible. It's important that they be gentle because people who are ADD and creative are also sensitive, and you don't need to be hit over the head with a brick in order to get a lesson. Nothing is to be gained by the proverbial "no pain, no gain" approach. That is simply an excuse by the teacher or mentor to utilize brute-force tactics that serve his purposes, not the purposes of the student.

It's also important that your mentor or group be positive. If you have issues involving trust, that means you have been hurt already. You need support and positive thinking in order to risk taking a chance to let your precious creativity out one more time. Your mentor also needs to be flexible because the style of brain wiring that you have is likely to be different from the mainstream. The mentor must not be wed to "This is the way that things must be done," or, "This is the *right* way," or "the only way." Remember, this is an exercise in rebuilding trust, so you want to have all the help you can get.

Your mentor or group could help you find an appropriate place to show off your creative endeavors in a safe setting. Maybe that would be a performing-arts presentation or neighborhood art show. Perhaps the group will help you find an appropriate magazine to send your poetry to. You will feel supported and nurtured by any of these opportunities.

After gaining support from a mentor or small group, reach out for nurturing from a friend. Again chose wisely so that you are likely to meet with success, getting what you need. Tell your friend that you are learning to build trust and would like for that person to be your special support system for a while. Ask that person to tell you what a fine job you are doing or give you other words of encouragement. Maybe you would like to get a hug from the friend when you tell of something creative you've just finished. Remember, nurturing the release of your creativity is the goal.

Finally, you come to the stage of self-nurturing. Don't rush into this stage because it is the last one. Sometimes adults who have not had much nurturing try to do it for themselves and want to take this step first. If you feel too afraid to reach out then naturally, be self-nurturing until you have grown strong enough to try trusting someone else with your creative life. But in the natural unfolding process that children go through, self-nurturing comes much later than the other two forms.

Saying nice things to yourself is one way to be self-nurturing. Doing a creative job and then treating yourself to a reward is another. You might give yourself permission to get a massage, have an ice cream sundae, go for a bike ride, or any of a number of other things. Pick something that will make you feel good and tell yourself that you deserve to be cared for in this way and that you will nurture yourself anytime you want.

Each of these exercises helps build your trust. Don't be surprised if it is hard to learn to trust. After all, trust is the most basic, first step to becoming a whole, happy, healthy, courageous person who can own your creativity and risk exposing it for others to enjoy. Be gentle with yourself but don't quit—except to take a breather now and again. That way you can learn to trust that you will not again abandon the creative aspects of yourself.

Identity

Unleashing the second Core Component of Human Nature means you turn your attention to your creative identity. You may know a lot about yourself intellectually, physically, and emotionally, but this is the time to take a close look at the creative aspect of who you are.

Your creative identity came as a part of your initial software. You didn't make it up then, and you won't make it up now. You can't buy it. It's a free gift. But you may have buried it or purposely put it aside for a period of time. Pay attention to discovering your creative identity now and you can retain it forever.

EXERCISE 1. Fill in the following blank:

Creatively, I express myself _____

_____

The question here is not whether or not you are creative but how you express your creativity. If you have trouble filling this out yourself, ask a friend or family member to help you. When they tell you something, don't deny it. Write what they say down.

Here are a few suggestions to get your thinking going. Does your creativity show itself through an art, craft, or through music? Are you a creative thinker, problem-solver, builder, cook, or driver? Did you create a new business? Are you creative in the kinds of trouble you get into? Are you creative in the way in which you have brought chaos into your life? Have you followed the straight and narrow or have you made decisions for yourself, perhaps in a creative way?

EXERCISE 2. Find the natural creative you. Currently you may or may not be expressing yourself creatively in a way that fits you. As you pay closer attention to how you feel, you will know whether or not something fits you. Then you'll get in touch with the natural you. To get on track, you must live authentically. If you've not thought about yourself and your inherent likes and dislikes, it may seem difficult to know where to start. To help you, let's look at what you favor. Fill in these blanks by listing your most and least favorite.

Art form _____

Type of music _____

Sculpture medium _____

Performing art _____

Style of clothing _____

Style of home _____

Style of interior decoration _____

Way to spend free time   _____

Way to solve problems _____

Way to express your creativity _____

Now describe:

The most fantastic invention you can imagine _____

_____

An imaginary mode of transportation _____

_____

The silliest thing you can think of to do _____

_____

The wackiest dream you can imagine_____

_____

Exercise 3. List at least five creative people you admire and explain why you admire them.

_____

_____

_____

_____

_____

EXERCISE 4. Just how self-aware can you become? Let's take time now to further develop your self-awareness. The following exercises will help you heighten your perceptions. You have five senses that you are commonly aware of: sight, hearing, smell, taste, and touch. In addition, you have a strong intuitive sense as a person who is creative and ADD. With a little practice you can become more sensitive in each of these areas. Your mind will experience the attention to these senses as validation and permission that it's okay for them to operate.

Sight: For five minutes (or three if you get restless easily), look at something familiar that is near you. For example, you may wish to survey the ceiling of the room you are in. Or perhaps study the back of your hand or a piece of jewelry that attracts you. Look at the object from different angles and in different lights. Note its texture, size, color, shading, and shape. You are likely to notice aspects that you never saw before.

Hearing: Stop right now and concentrate on what you hear. You may want to shut your eyes—your sense of hearing will become more acute this way. Maybe you hear the hum of your computer when you consciously pay attention to it. Then suddenly you become aware of a car driving down the street. Perhaps the motor sounds like it needs a tune-up. Listen for several minutes. You'll probably be surprised at what goes on around you.

Smell: Take a piece of food such as an apple slice. Hold it close to your nose and smell it. Again, you may wish to shut your eyes. Your sense of smell is delicate and tends to wear out fast, so concentrate on the first few whiffs. On the first inhalation pay particular attention to memories that come to your mind. What feelings are stirred by the aroma? Can you smell the moisture or dryness of the food?

Taste: Now taste a piece of food. A nut, fruit slice, or piece of cereal works well for this. Start by licking the food. Try shutting your eyes during part of this exercise for greater clarity. Next, hold a bit of the food in your mouth, rolling it around. Your sense of touch will tend to give you feedback about the piece of food in your mouth, but remember to also taste it. Pay attention to the stimulation you get from the food. You'll probably notice that your sense of smell provides you with information during the taste exercise. Try to sort each stimulus out from the others. Finally, begin to chew the food. Pay attention to the taste released through this process. What do you notice that you did not notice earlier?

Touch: Take an object in your hand. Or you may want to use your hand or forearm as the site of your investigation. At first, shut your eyes. Run your fingers over the object. Then run your fingernail over it. Tap it lightly. Simply become acquainted with it through your sense of touch.

These five senses commonly convey information to us on a daily basis. But there seems also to be a less well-understood sixth sense that some people trust more than any of the others. As someone who is ADD and creative, you are likely to have a great capacity for this sixth sense. It is sometimes called gut-level feeling and can be described as an inner knowing. Simply give yourself permission to develop this sense. Pay attention to tensions that come into your body such as a knot in your stomach when something is wrong or a warm flush across your face when something is right. Experiment by paying attention to whether you feel good or bad about something. Keep track of the results after you get a gut-level feeling and see what happens, depending on whether you felt good or bad. I bet you'll see a pattern soon.

> EXERCISE 5. Be a hedonist for a day. Take a day to go anywhere you want. See what you're drawn to. Tell your family and friends that you are unavailable. Go to a museum, an art store, a computer store, the library, the beach, or wherever you're drawn. Watch what attracts you. Notice how you feel and the level of intensity that you feel it. Maybe in the library you're attracted to a section with books about scientific inventions. Or maybe your eye rapidly passes that area of the stacks and seeks books on architecture. Browse with awareness.

For a second day give yourself permission to do or make anything you want. Get the supplies that you need ahead of time and go to it. Don't particularly try to make an end product, though you may if you wish. Concentrate on exploring and experimenting. Above all, have fun and be aware of what you enjoy.

Do as many of these exercises as you're drawn to and be aware that you are learning about your creative identity. Remember, creativity does not just mean arts-and-crafts creativity. Let yourself explore in any way that you want and rejoice in what pleases you.

Your Sense of Competence

To strengthen your sense of competence, your confidence in your creativity, let's first take a hard look at the processes that go into the construction of that confidence: experiencing, experimentation, expressiveness, and expansion. Each of these provides opportunities from which you can acquire self-confidence easily and fully, just as you could have as a child in a supportive environment. Each process come from a different perspective than the others. Each adds to the others so that, in the end, they work together to provide you with full-fledged, whole self-confidence in your abilities. With that sense of competence you can do whatever you want to do.

EXERCISE 1. Experiencing stems from natural curiosity that is the outgrowth of your fine intelligence. I encourage you to be aware of the six senses you worked with as you reconnected with your identity. Time spent with each provides opportunity from which to acquire self-confidence easily and fully. The curiosity to experience is innate—an offshoot of intelligence. Just give yourself permission to experience everything you do, now, and you will open a magical door to your creativity. Learn to live in the present. Fantasy is wonderful, but it can get in the way of your awareness. It carries you away from the present and may affect your ability to perform competently *now*.

So stop! What is happening around you right now? Check your five senses. Check your sixth sense. Check your goals. Check your behavior. Do your goals and behavior match? If not, what's off?

Now get an overview of what you are presently experiencing by looking at your answers to all of the above questions. This is the *now* in which you are living.

EXERCISE 2. Experimenting is the outgrowth of experiencing. By doing, you learn what works and what doesn't. You create a database from which you can later draw—the very raw materials of creativity are stored in it. You'll come to know the parameters of materials and experiences of all kinds by simply mentally logging their limitations and capabilities. It doesn't matter whether you are working with materials, personalities, or relationships. You will be able, later, to use what you've learned to create anything of interest to you.

To become comfortable trying new things, take the following steps. You may want to ask a buddy to help you. Be sure that you are trying something that *you* really *want* to do, not something you think you *ought* to do.

Step 1. Decide on a project you want to try or a skill you want to develop. Keep it simple. For example, rather than putting on a big dinner party for twenty people, try having three friends over for dessert.

Step 2. Make a plan ahead of time so you are clear about your goal, what you want to achieve, and how you want to accomplish it. Tell your buddy and ask for suggestions if you want them. If you prefer to work alone, do so.

Step 3. Follow through with your project. Remember, everything doesn't have to be perfect. You are simply trying to get used to trying something new.

Step 4. Congratulate yourself on all the good things you accomplished. Look for them and list them.

Step 5. Note the areas that you would like to improve. If you are on target with your learning, you will have made some errors that you would like to correct the next time. Remember, that's how you learn—by making errors and analyzing them.

Step 6. Congratulate yourself on discovering some further learning opportunities.

EXERCISE 3. Part of building your self-confidence, and ultimately your sense of competence, includes increasing your ability to be expressive. Your own body is a primary tool for communicating this expressiveness. That body needs to be in topnotch form.

You will need to pay particular attention to breathing deeply and thoroughly, feeding your body with the energy that comes from having sufficient oxygen. Right now, try breathing more deeply than you have been. Dip down to the bottom of your diaphragm. Fill your lungs with air. Hold the air for four counts, and then release it slowly, smoothly, and completely. Repeat the exercise for several minutes two or three times a day for five days.

You will find yourself relaxing much of the tension inside you, allowing you to experience the world more freely. You will discover a clearer awareness of everything around you. You may want to say to yourself as you exhale "the tension within me leaves as I breathe out."

To further free yourself, turn your attention to your body, with all its muscles and joints. When was the last time you stretched? Lie down on a firm surface and stretch all over from head to toe. Slowly raise your arms, turn your head back and forth, and pull yourself to the right and left. Try pointing your toes as you do this. Then relax them. You may be surprised to hear your joints snapping and crackling. Just move slowly and gently, and you won't hurt yourself.

Nature provides many opportunities to extend your ability to be expressive. Wiggle your toes in the sand, make angels-in-the-snow, squeeze mud through your fingers and toes. Write in the mud, make mud pies and mud bombs and mud paintings.

Try making faces in the mirror to see how expressive you can be. Make a happy face, then a sad one, a mad one, and a silly one.

Finally do the "rag doll" exercise. Stand with your knees bent, relaxed. Let your arms dangle at your sides. Gently bounce up and down, raising your heels off the ground. Hang loose. Add music if you want and let your body go.

Notice as you do these expression-building exercises that you become increasingly comfortable with yourself. The ability to freely express yourself pushes the boundaries of your creativity way out, releasing you to be who you were always meant to be.

EXERCISE 4. The expansion of what you've learned so far also builds self-confidence, because you take what you've achieved and carry it further. Through flexing your muscles you'll find the outer limits of what you can do. You are likely to find that those limits are initially broader than you might have expected. Even more exciting, the more you work with expansion, the more the limits keep expanding.

Take any of the previous exercises and do more than you did the first time. For example, as you stretched before, do so again now. This time do more than you did before. Then let your body slowly relax, and then stretch beyond the limits you imagined possible. Expand your possibilities and capabilities, but don't use force.

EXERCISE 5. Learn to make mistakes. Most people are afraid of making mistakes. Where does this come from? Maybe from those frightening red marks on school papers or chastisements from parents and others. But I ask you to think about mistakes in a new way—as guideposts for learning. Use them to make changes in direction with regard to whatever you are doing.

Here's the Mistake-A-Day exercise.
Step 1. Carry a notepad around with you. Each day for a week write down one mistake that you made that day.
Step 2. After acknowledging your error, decide what you want to do to fix it rather than apologize for it.
Step 3. Implement the remedy you have decided on.
Step 4. Consider what went into making the mistake in the first place.
Step 5. Congratulate yourself on having repaired your mistake and taken steps toward preventing a repetition of the error in the future.
Step 6. Continue noting a mistake a day for the duration of the week. This will help desensitize you to the making of mistakes and will allow you to become much freer and creatively more expressive.
Each of the exercises in this section will help you become more confident, building your sense of competence. Remember, this core component has to do with *feeling* competent. It has little to do with outside judgments or standards about how you do things. By wanting to be competent and believing you are competent, you become competent. From this feeling, creativity becomes possible. You can then become as creatively expressive as you wish.

A Sense of Emotional Power
When you were very, very young, you had to rely on someone else to meet your

needs, and then the time came when you wanted to meet them yourself. You wanted to be in charge of yourself. That's what the sense of emotional power is all about.

But emotional power is a two-edged sword. Just as a fire is wonderful when contained within a fireplace or furnace, so, too, must emotional power be contained within limits. Generally, the society in which you live will clearly define those limits. If you work within those limits, you will be considered a socialized, healthy person.

Emotional power allows you to take responsibility to get or do what you want and to reach your creative goals. Though the sense of competence motivates you, the sense of emotional power drives the engine of your productions. It supplies the energy to actually get something done, rather than just dream about it.

EXERCISE 1. Clean up your environment. In order to build your emotional power, you have to live and work in an emotionally supportive environment. If someone or something is abusing you, pulling you down, or having a continuously negative effect on you, you need to consider removing yourself from that environment or else seeing that the abusive factor is removed. No one can—or should—get used to being abused.

This abuse may come in the form of a person who verbally tells you that your creations are "stupid" or a "waste of time." Or it could be could be a dirty or polluted workroom. Either way you and your creativity are being compromised.

EXERCISE 2. Give yourself permission to do what you want to do. Become aware of the difference between "I *should* do . . ." and "I *want* to do . . . " Give yourself permission to follow what you *want*. Become aware of people in your environment who tell you that you *should* do such and such. Give yourself permission to say, "Thank you for your suggestion. I will consider it." Then give yourself permission to do what you *want* and feel is in your best interest as well as the best interest of all concerned.

You have now taken charge of getting your own needs met. That is being responsible. You are acting as an emotionally powerful person.

EXERCISE 3. Set your own limits. The key to building your emotional power is your ability to set and maintain your limits. Basically, limits define what you will and will not allow to happen to you. This week take one new situation in your life and apply some limit.

Here's how to go about applying those limits. First of all, listen to how you feel in the following situation. Suppose someone asks or tells you to do something that you really don't want to do or don't have the time to do. Say to the person, "I can't possibly help you now." If you want to, you can say, "Feel free to ask me in the future. Maybe I can help you then." If you never want the person to approach you again, say, "I'm not willing to be involved in that, even at a later time."

EXERCISE 4. Learn to say no. When you are asked to do something you don't like or want to do, say no. You don't have to be offensive about it. You can say, "I really can't let myself add anything more to my list of things to do right now." Or you might want to say, "There's nothing wrong with your asking me to be involved, but I'm simply am not willing to participate at this time." Above all do not make long excuses and do not lie. Don't say your Aunt Matilda is sick, and you have to visit when, in fact, you have no Aunt Matilda. Face the situation in a straightforward manner and just say no.

EXERCISE 5. Use your body to build emotional power. Walk with your head high, stand tall, and let your arms swing easily at your sides while your legs take longer strides than usual. Feel proud of how you look and show yourself off with pride. That doesn't mean going around with your nose in the air. Keep it level with the ground but broadcast, "World, here I come."

Shake hands firmly. Ever shaken a hand that feels like a limp fish? Remember how you felt about that person? Though you don't need to overpower the other person as if you were a sumo wrestler, grip the other person's hand firmly, physically stating that you have substance, and you are not afraid to meet him or her.

EXERCISE 6. Use sports and activities to build emotional power. Certain sports will help you learn to be assertive, which is a major component of emotional power. Racquetball is one of them. Any sport that demands that you charge or contest for position in order to score builds your sense of power. Additional examples include soccer, basketball, and football, and there are many others. Choose one that you are drawn to.

Horseback riding also is a great teacher of power. You *must* be in charge of the horse or it will "take you for a ride." That doesn't mean you have to be cruel or abusive which, unfortunately, some people confuse with being powerful. An animal senses whether we are sure of ourselves or afraid. It is true, I promise you.

EXERCISE 7. Develop your own personalized slogans. All of us have heard phrases that make us stop and think because we know they apply to our own lives. Which phrases or slogans work best for you? Which ones help support your personal goals? Write them down on sticky notes or cards and put them on the bathroom mirror, refrigerator, car dashboard, or in your wallet. That way you'll see them many times during the day and they will become a habitual way of thinking about yourself.

Here are some examples you can consider—and there are many, many others.

> *Say what you really feel.*
> *Do what feels right!*
> *Take full responsibility for your actions.*
> *Go for the gold!*
> *Act, don't talk.*
> *Set your limits.*

Self-Control

The first four Core Components of Human Nature—trust, identity, competence and power—lead people to become responsible, motivated, and trustworthy, with a firm grasp on their identity. With this foundation in place a person can be counted on to learn to control himself, rather than being controlled by threats, guilt, or force. People who have that foundation in place automatically want to do what is right for themselves and others. That is what I mean by self-control.

This core component reflects whether you do things because of an outside force (because you feel you *should* do something) or because you have your own values and want to live by them doing what you *want*. When you do something because you *should* do it, rather than because you *want* to do it—like majoring in accounting in college because your parents told you you should, instead of majoring in art because you wanted to—you end up feeling resentment. Not doing something you *should* do but don't *want* to leads to guilt. Either way you lose.

For you to be in personal control of yourself and your life, you must act based on decisions that you personally believe in and want to do.

EXERCISE. Changing "shoulds" to "wants." Start off by thinking about any job you are faced with in the very near future. Then ask yourself honestly whether or not you *want* to do the job. If your answer is no, ask yourself whether you would be willing to look for an alternative. If you are willing to look for another option, make a list of several alternatives you can think of. On your list, you might want to include hiring someone else to do the job, making a trade, or simply saying no. Then consider the alternatives and decide which one you will implement.

Now you can be in control of yourself and your decision and not end up feeling guilty or resentful because you let others determine what you do. You still have values, but they are your own, and you use your thinking mind to propel yourself into action.

FINDING A SAFE ENVIRONMENT FOR YOUR CREATIVITY

Now that you've reconnected with your natural creativity by doing these exercises, you need to find a safe environment for your creativity so that you can explore it and use it. Then you won't find yourself separated from your creativity again.

A Safe Learning Environment

As you already know, building a safe environment so that you can develop trust is important. But I want to underscore how very important that is as you begin to let your vulnerable, sensitive, wonderful creativity out. Because you are just now learning to trust and feel secure as a creative person, I want you to go slowly and feel sure that the results will feel good for you.

Finding a safe and nurturing learning environment for your creativity means that you avoid working with someone who is constantly criticizing you or your creative product. As we've discussed earlier, many people believe that pain must be endured if progress is to be made and the student is to toughen up. They believe that being harshly criticized is one of the ways that pain is transmitted to a student or novice.

I see no reason to continue to project this myth. Training and teaching do not require that you be berated with what is *wrong* with you or your work. Rather, a healthy, knowledgeable teacher will simply say what is right about what you have done and then show you some alternative ways to handle what's not working in your best interest.

Particularly in the arena of creativity, there are few rights and wrongs. It is very important for you to remember this. Design and style are matters of personal preference. Your idea is as good as anybody else's.

The tangible building of skills, of course, requires certain practice. In this arena, a good teacher can show you what has worked previously, and you can try it. You can take the elements that you want and, being creative, experiment beyond them.

Anyone who puts you or your work down, tells you that you don't have talent or in any other way abuses you is not a right and proper teacher for someone who is sensitive. Don't buy into the idea that you have to go through torture to achieve your goal. Severe criticism is no way to coax creativity out.

Finding your Fit

Finding your fit means doing things in a way that is natural for you and best uses your particular array of talents, gifts, and interests. For example, if you are tall and sturdily built and slow on your feet you might fit better into the job required of an offensive lineman than that of a running back.

If you like to work with your hands and can even close your eyes and feel what you want to make, sculpture would be a good fit for you. If, however, you don't much like getting your hands gooey and you prefer to work visually, you would find a better fit as a photographer than a sculptor.

When you find your fit, you feel *right, easy* about what you're doing. Learning tends to come easily and you will tend to have a skill in that area. That's how you'll know if you've found your fit.

You must find your fit to place yourself in a safe environment to let your creativity blossom. Trying to work in a way that doesn't fit creates tension, requires you to use extra energy, and erodes your efficiency and effectiveness. You are much less likely to succeed and are likely to become tired and stressed from what you do. That is not constructive. To maximize your skills you want to work within your own personal range of capability and fit.

For example, consider Sid. Sid, who has a degree in marketing, was given the job of writing copy for an advertising agency. He almost quit his job over that one assignment. It's not that he didn't try. He did. But he just could not get the words to come out right. He began to wonder if maybe he'd majored in the wrong field in college. Yet he'd had a dream of designing campaigns that would sell products or services. He'd thought he could do it.

When he talked to a friend about what he should do, the friend made an interesting observation. "You know, Sid, when you were in school, you always hated the writing part of your assignments," the friend said. "I remember your complaining.

I do remember, though, that you loved creating video campaigns. I think you are much more of a visual designer than someone who creates with words."

Instantly, Sid felt relief. He knew his friend was right. He'd taken the writing job to get a start with the agency, but it was all wrong for him. The job simply didn't fit him.

Now that he had that understanding of himself, Sid was faced with a decision. He could: 1) weather out the current situation while waiting for another job to open up, 2) go to his boss and explain his situation and ask for a transfer within the company, 3) actively look for another job that fit him better with another company, or 4) go into business for himself. Though there were pros and cons to each of these options, he knew one thing. He had to get into a job situation that fit him better—and soon.

And then there was Vickey. Vickey lived a very creative lifestyle. She didn't have one specific talent that shown brightly, but everything she did or touched carried her individual creative flair. When she wasn't pleased with her local school, she decided to home school her kids. When her husband needed to keep track of his sales figures, she designed a system that worked for him to keep the books in order. Later, when the kids were older and the family needed money, she looked at her options and decided she liked to cook and wanted to have her own cafe. She worked for someone for a year first to get the hang of running her own business and then set off on her own.

On the first anniversary of her cafe's opening, Vickey reflected on the year and her life in general. She realized that she had truly found her fit with the cafe business. She loved it. It utilized the many skills that she'd built—good relations with people, her ability to design systems and keep track of finances, and her talent for creating food that people enjoyed. She also loved the ambience that made her cafe the gathering place for creative people in her community.

All in all Vickey's happiness stemmed from her having found her fit. Through the previous experiences that she's had, she realized that she'd been sorting through what she liked and didn't like for years. Though she hadn't consciously or purposely monitored what she liked to do or didn't like, she had paid attention to these factors along the way. Neither did she realize she was looking for her fit, but she was. Because of that, she found it and became a happy person who loves what she does.

WHO MEASURES THE VALUE OF YOUR CREATIVITY?

Once you've brought your creativity safely out into the world, it will be open to judgment, some of which will feel good and some of which will not feel so good.

I am going to give you some suggestions for protecting yourself, so that you and your creativity can stay safe and secure and not have to retreat for protection.

The most important lesson you can learn is to measure the value of your creativity yourself. Think about that for a minute: measure the value of your creativity yourself. Don't turn that right over to someone else. You alone understand and know the total value of your creativity and your creative products. It is especially important to realize this immediately after you've coaxed your creativity out into the open.

But don't fool yourself or believe everything you hear about visibly successful people when they are criticized. Though they may say, "Oh, I've learned to be tough and not let criticism or judgment bother me," I've never gotten close to such a person's inner feelings without finding that, in fact, they are bothered. Their tough exterior is a form of protection to talk themselves and others into not feeling so bad when the affronts come. But underneath, they are sensitive—just like you are.

When you leave the measurement of your work up to someone else, you give your power away to that other person. You don't know whether that person is able to give praise, is jealous, can look objectively at your work, or hates the general form of your work no matter who produces it.

For example, Hillary began to write poetry a few months ago, and she wanted to share what she'd written with a friend. So, tentatively, she asked her friend whether or not she would listen. Half-heartedly, her friend said she would. So Hillary read a couple of poems to her. But her friend said little and didn't compliment or support her, and Hillary put her things away after having read just a few poems.

Devastated, Hillary didn't ask anyone else to listen to her poetry for some time. When she finally took the risk, her new listener affirmed her productions. She asked questions about the subject of the poems, which told Hillary that she'd actually listened. Her new listener even made comments about how much she liked the analogies that Hillary used.

At that point, Hillary told her what had happened earlier when she had read her poems to a friend. She found out that her first friend just didn't like poetry. It wasn't Hillary's poetry that caused the lack of response. It was the limitations of her friend.

Hillary had allowed herself to be devastated because she had looked for affirmation from outside of herself. What Hillary needed to work on was her own judgment of her own work. She could ask herself whether or not her poem accomplished the goal she had set. Did she say what she wanted to say? Was she pleased with how she crafted her poem? How could she make it sound better to her? Did she feel any twinges that told her she might want to consider changing some aspect of her poem, or was she satisfied with it as it stood?

Hillary must come to believe in her own work—whether others accept it or not. Ironically, the more she believes in her own work, the more others will support her. That's often how this evaluation of creative work goes.

So how do you measure the worth of your own creativity? Here's a list of questions you can ask yourself.

1. *Have I done the best I can do?* If you have to ask someone else whether or not what you've done is good, then you don't understand the structure of your own work. The integrity of your work comes from what *you* wanted it to be. Once you've worked hard to attain the highest quality of work you can, you have to know that the quality is good. That's what you use to measure it—the fact that it's the highest quality you can produce at that time.

2. *Do I feel personal satisfaction from what I've created?* Do you enjoy looking at, reading, or considering your own work? Does it continue to give you pleasure? And be sure to consider the difference between Do I like the work? and will other people like it?

3. *Have I accomplished what I set out to do?* If the act of using your creativity has brought you personal satisfaction, then that's one way of measuring the success of your creativity or your creative product. If you really love what you've done and really enjoyed doing it, then that's that!

Personal satisfaction is not necessarily related to what's popular. When you are extremely creative, you will probably find that you are ahead of the market. What a lot of other people like may be less experimental and more staid than what you produce. Know that your lack of popularity now may change later on when others catch up and "get" what you are doing or saying.

A Look Toward the Future

Later, after you've coaxed your creativity out of hiding and learned to enjoy it again and become comfortable with it yourself again, then you might want someone else involved in judging, editing, or molding your product to help you improve it. Once you can do that, it's really pretty exciting and may take you to a new level.

As my own vulnerable, creative self has been emerging, I've done all the things I've been sharing with you. I began to truly believe that I could also write poetry, short stories, and performing-arts pieces. My belief empowered me to reach out, seeking a new level of expression. So I consulted with a musician friend of mine and a playwright friend. My questions to each were, How can I make this better? What will showcase this work so that viewers and readers feel the excitement I feel writing them?

Even as I asked the questions, my stomach tightened. I was afraid—but afraid of what? The part of me that is sensitive and holds the childlike vulnerability of my creative talent still wanted assurance. After all, I was risking reaching out to others rather than simply enfolding my vulnerable part in my own arms.

However, I had chosen my potential critics carefully, and they didn't let me down. Each made structural suggestions, saying in essence, I can visualize your work this way. How does that feel to you? Neither put my work down nor told me emphatically how it should be. Humbly, they made *suggestions*. I could take the suggestions or leave them. I wasn't robbed of my power.

The reality was that their suggestions were magnificent. I had not thought of them myself and probably never would have. Suddenly I had a new feeling. My creative work had stimulated still another creation. Through teamwork, started by my original production, we reached a new level. The final product was better than what I could have created on my own. But that final product would never have come into being if I hadn't done my initial writing.

I became a part of a creative team. Let me tell you, that felt great. Now I'm hooked. Not only did it not hurt, but now I *love* teaming with others. The end result is more than any of us could create individually. What a thrill!

Creative collaboration can be something very exciting—and something for you to look forward to in the future.

WHAT IF YOUR REINSTATED CREATIVITY GOES UNRECOGNIZED BY OTHERS

But what happens to you if your creativity goes unrecognized by others? How do you live with that?

If your work isn't recognized, you need to recognize that as a temporary situation in relation to the environment you're in at the time. To be sure, sometimes it takes years to be recognized. But don't quit—unless you want to. You may need to find a better environment, to find your fit. Keep your eyes open for an environment in which you'll enjoy exposing your creativity.

When it comes to what you can do with your unrecognized creative endeavors, I'd advise that you not throw them away. They are precious and you are their keeper. It's up to you to take good care of them. After all, they wouldn't have come through you unless they were valuable and important in the first place.

Put them in a safe place and do something else for a while. After all, you may just need to wait until others catch up with you and are ready for what you have to contribute. History is full of inventions and creations that were ahead of their time. The trick is to stay aware and take care of yourself and your creativity emotionally. You have breathed life into your project. You must continue to have positive thoughts about it.

I know what that's like, because that's what happened to me when I developed the concept of the Core Components of Human Nature.

When I first began to observe small children in the early 1970s, I quickly realized that I was viewing some building blocks of human nature that were not written about in the way I was seeing them. I spent several years continuing my observation and working on a new framework of human behavior that has come to be known as the Core Components of Human Nature.

Although the five components were easy for me to talk about to groups and people understood them quickly, it has taken twenty-five years for the time to be right for more wide-spread dissemination of the theory. Many times I was discouraged as I tried to show people the implications of the Core Components for business, family life, and relationships in general.

Meanwhile, the inner-child and self-help movements have led people to want to know why we people are the way we are. The Core Components theory provides a major answer, and people are now becoming interested in it. I can't say that I don't wish all of this had come together sooner. I'd be lying to say anything different. But I am glad the time is now. And I know that timing is everything. Perhaps if the Core Components had been prematurely understood, it would have suffered an early death, unsupported by groundwork that needed to be completed first.

There is little I or anyone else can do to push time or readiness, however. So while you're waiting, say your prayers, keep your eyes open, and be ready to support your creative efforts, whatever they are — regardless of whether or not you are receiving affirmation right now. Your time will come.

I welcome the reinstatement of your creativity. Enjoy it.

chapter**nine**

Learning and Creativity for the ADD Individual

W HAT DOES the word learning mean to you? When you hear that word, does your stomach immediately tighten up? Do you start to sweat? How do you feel about having to prove that you've learned something? Does your throat constrict or your mouth get dry? Those are common physical reactions in someone with ADD—someone who has tried for years to squeeze into an educational system that just didn't fit. For that person, learning is a term often associated with struggle, frustration, failure, and humiliation.

Yet, if you take a step back and think about what learning really means, you'll find learning only means letting in some new information or experience, or letting something new out, such as a new thought or understanding that comes from synthesizing information.

To do this—to learn—you must open yourself up to change. In order to be open to change, you must feel secure that you will be able to understand new material when faced with a learning opportunity. You also need to feel secure in expressing yourself and in sharing your perspective of what has been learned.

If you find a discrepancy between how you feel about learning and what it takes to truly learn, then you are among the majority of people with ADD who have developed a fear of learning situations, yet crave to learn. Like all the others, you were eager to learn until you got hurt in the process—by age five or six, or even earlier.

Learning is a creative act. You must release old limitations so you can open yourself up to new experiences. To be a truly receptive learner, you have to be willing to see things in new ways. In fact, you are actually changing the world from the way you previously knew it.

Remember how you visualized the world as a young child? You probably thought of the whole world in terms of your family or your neighborhood. If you traveled to Grandma's house in the country, you came to realize that the world included areas that were different from the one in which you lived. But unless you were reared in a family of world travelers, you would have been about nine or ten years old before you learned about the great variety of cultures, peoples, and places in this world. Learning about Africa, Europe, and South America in school would have changed your perception of the world, and changed it drastically.

At that time you might have begun to realize that some people cooked food differently than your family did and that the clothing some people wore was very different from what you wore. You might have begun to realize that there were many, many languages spoken in the world—not just English and the one or two other languages you had heard—and that even children are fluent in languages with sounds you couldn't even wrap your tongue around.

You became a different person the day you began to learn all this in school. Of course, much of you was still the same. But your view of the world, and your place in it, had permanently changed. It's really quite amazing, isn't it?

So, as you see, learning creates a different you. Learning is a creative process, and creativity is a learning process. They walk hand in hand. You can't have one without the other. To create, you must open yourself to new experiences. You must draw from your environment. But if you have already closed yourself off to learning, you have also inadvertently closed yourself off to creativity.

The creative process is about eliminating boundaries—previously held perceptions and limitations about how something looks, functions, or *should* be. For any of us to let our boundaries down, we must take a risk. To take that risk, we need to feel secure.

Think of a time when you took such a risk and tried something new. Recall how you felt before and after you let your boundaries down. Was it a good experience or a bad one for you? What did you learn? At best, you learned what you intended to learn. If your learning was relatively pain free, you would have come away with a sense of the joy of learning. If you suffered embarrassment or anxiety or the job was just beyond your capability at that time, you would have come away from the experience with a painful memory. Even though we often forget specific incidents after we've grown up, we remember that learning is not fun. Those negative feelings make us feel vulnerable when we are in a learning situation.

TRADITIONAL EDUCATION VS. TRAINING

There are two very different ways to learn something new. You can be taught *about* something by being lectured to or by reading about it. Or you can be trained in a hands-on way, including tasks, skills, and even thought processes.

Neither method is better than the other. They are just different.

In traditional education students are generally taught *about* something. The teacher talks or the student is referred to a book or worksheet or occasionally an audio tape or computer. As the student progresses in school, he also is required to learn about the theory behind the subject he is studying.

For example, in learning to be a counselor students are often taught about the predominant theories of the time—psychological, human nature, and human pathology. This information doesn't actually teach anyone *how* to counsel. But teachers believe that this information explains why clients/patients act the way they do, why people counsel the way they do, and the effects that counseling is supposed to have on a client/patient.

But there is a step missing here. With this type of education, it is very possible for a student to understand the information presented and still not have a clue about how to apply that information. On the other hand a student may not be able to repeat the theoretical material back on a test, but she may understand and be able to apply the concepts in real life.

People who are ADD tend to need hands-on experience in order to learn. *Show* me, don't *tell* me about something. Or, worse yet, don't tell me to just read about it. That's even one step farther removed from the hands-on experience. Just let me get in there and work with the situation. Instead of a traditional teaching relationship, give me a mentor, give me a demonstration. The apprenticeship method of teaching works much better for people who are ADD than the traditional teaching we find in our schools today.

Similarly, creative people are also prone to be hands-on kinesthetic learners who want to experiment themselves to see what works and why, rather than be told the *right* way of doing something. Creative learning utilizes trial-and-error experience to maximum effect.

For example, when Gilberto bought a computer recently, he pulled the manual out of the box and looked at it. He knew he *should* read it first, but he felt that would be a waste of time. Nevertheless, feeling guilty, he started to read it and tried as hard as he could to follow the directions. An hour later, he knew no more than he had previously. But his head hurt, and he felt frustrated and stupid. Once again, he felt like a failure trying to figure out what the written word was telling him to do.

He was tempted to just take the computer back to the store and give up on it when a friend called and offered to come by and show him a few things. As a last resort, Gilberto agreed, but he prepared to be frustrated again. He figured that the computer was just too much for him to learn. He trusted that his friend wouldn't make fun of him. But all his previous learning experiences taught him that he wouldn't be able to learn something as complicated as a computer.

To his surprise, with his friend showing him what to do and then having him do it, Gilberto quickly learned how to do simple things with his computer. He was thrilled as he felt a new sense of knowledge in an area that he had thought was unavailable to him. His friend agreed to continue to help him from time to time. Gilberto was on his way to the development of a new skill.

It was never true that Gilberto was not intelligent enough to learn how to use a computer. It was just that Gilberto couldn't learn how to use a computer by *reading* about it. He needed to be *shown* what to do and why, and to be given the opportunity to get in there and try it for himself. Gilberto didn't need to be *taught*—he needed to be *trained*.

Training is a hands-on approach to learning, and the old apprenticeship model is based on it. Training allows someone to learn something through a hands-on, repetitive approach. Questions are encouraged all along the way—especially questions about how something works and why it works the way it does.

In the apprenticeship model the student isn't just reading or hearing about the subject he wants to learn about. Instead, he is slowly indoctrinated into the actual skills that are needed. Those skills can be physical or mental.

A few professions today utilize this kind of hands-on approach. For example, if you want to become a chef, you have to work in a kitchen and serve under a chef. No one expects you to learn to cook by simply reading about it. You have to learn to use your senses to feel the texture of the dough, see when pastry is ready, or taste the right blend of spices.

Physicians, counselors, and teachers are required to serve internships, to get hands-on experience. Unfortunately, however, these internships are preceded by a lot of book learning. Although they might do very well in those professions, people who need a hands-on learning style probably wouldn't pass enough of the book material to make it to the hands-on part of the education.

Ironically, many people who need a hands-on style of education can better access the written word after they've had a kinesthetic learning experience. In the end, does it really matter which comes first?

TRAINING AND CREATIVITY

I'll never forget taking an art correspondence course when I was a young teenager. As I mentioned earlier, I had wanted very much to do artwork. So I signed up for the course and received my assignments and the booklets telling me how to learn certain drawing skills. The problem was that I couldn't *feel* what the words were trying to tell me. I did the best I could but I never got the feeling. I also never finished the course. I felt blocked from being an artist, relegating art to the category of hobby in my life. I couldn't be a "real" artist.

Creativity cannot be taught out of a book. Teaching a subject that is inherently creative—such as art, music, dance, engineering design, architecture—requires some form of mentorship that includes dialogue about the effects of trial-and-error experiences, and the student's feeling about his or her work and progress. That type of experience draws the student forward in the learning process. Affirmation of what works well, and clarification of what doesn't, guides a student to success in developing a new skill.

Training and creativity go together as the student takes one step at a time. The teacher of a creative skill might end up working harder than the student as he discovers how that student learns and analyzes what type of help the student needs. Together, through their relationship, the teacher and the student will "birth" the capability within the student, bringing it to light under the student's control.

Because creativity encourages experimentation and openness, a creative approach to learning fits people who are ADD. Similarly, because training encourages experimentation and openness, it fits people who are both ADD and creative better than book learning does. If book learning is required, having a hands-on learning experience before the books are opened helps make the written word more accessible.

Taking Lessons

I bought a piano when my kids were young: I wanted to expose them to as many interests as I could. A friend came over and sat down and started to run his fingers over the keys. Though he'd never played and didn't read music, he sat for more than an hour experimenting with the piano.

Noticing his interest, I said, "I bet you'd really enjoy taking piano lessons."

His response shocked me. "Oh, I don't want to take lessons," he said. "I'm enjoying what I'm doing."

At the time I argued with him. I tried to convince him that he *had* to take lessons if he wanted to play the piano. But finally, I heard what he was trying to tell me. "Lessons will get in my way of having an experience with the piano," he said. "What I want to do is to get to know the piano."

I've never forgotten the lesson I learned from my friend. I had been so indoctrinated with the fact that the only way to learn something was to take formal lessons, that it never occurred to me that someone could explore and experiment and learn for himself. Imagine—learning something by just fooling around with it!

I've seen adults and children turned off to many interests because of formal lessons. I recall when a school-age friend of my son's wanted to learn to play the drums. The instructor told the boy he had to learn to play the bells first because that's how percussion was taught at the school. Now, this boy didn't want to play the bells nor did he care to learn percussion. Rather, he felt a desire to play the drums. He was clear in his mind and heart. But since the teacher's position was non-negotiable, he chose not to play anything.

Personally, I have to admit I don't see much of a connection between bells and drums. They don't sound the same. Bells don't feel the same in my hand as drum sticks. They don't require the same approach to playing. But maybe the teacher needed someone to play the bells and already had too many students who wanted to play drums.

In all probability this incident did not change this child's life dramatically. But I know him now as an adult, and I know that playing music is not a part of his life. I cannot help but wonder whether he might have at least developed an interesting avocation if he'd been allowed to follow his interest and play the drums when he was ten.

Of course, lessons can help a person master a skill. Learning the tricks of the trade in creating a wash when painting with watercolors, or learning how to choose the right saw in carpentry could save a student a lot of time. But lessons in the "right" way to paint flowers or the "right" way to make a wooden puzzle can stifle a student's desire to explore and follow her own creative instincts.

Perhaps the most appropriate time to take lessons is when we are hungry for some information or knowledge that we haven't been able to find on our own. There are times when a few lessons can give a learner a head start in making better use of the materials or instruments at hand. But time to experiment on one's own is also very important. That time is hard to come by when there is material that must be learned before the next lesson.

If you are considering whether or not to take some lessons, think about your desires and goals. Here are a few questions you might want to ask yourself.

What am I really looking for by learning more in this particular area?

How do I want to use my new skills or abilities?

Am I doing this just for my own enjoyment?

Do I want to experiment to find the limits of my interest?

Do I want to develop this skill so I can use it repetitively?

Do I want to become more efficient with this skill?

Are there specific details or skills I want to learn so that I can get more enjoyment out of this interest? If so, what are those details or skills?

Could I learn those skills by experimenting on my own?

Would I like to be shown how to do something I can't do now?

As you review your answers, you will be able to discover whether or not lessons are the right thing for you now. Remember—there is no right or wrong answer. You just have to do what feels right to you as of now. If you choose not to take lessons, you can always start them later if you want to. If you do start lessons and they don't work out for you, you can always stop.

For example, let's suppose you are interested in ceramics. With the knowledge and skill you have right now, you can make a lot of different things for yourself. But suppose you want to be able to consistently produce high-quality work for sale. Or maybe you want to know how to create a certain type of glaze and, though you've been experimenting for a time, you haven't been able to produce the exact consistency you want. Perhaps you like the idea of being a part of a group that creates a certain style of pottery, and you want to learn how to make that type. If any of these apply to you, you may be ripe for lessons.

Your decision about whether or not to take lessons depends on what your goals for yourself are. I want to give you permission to self-teach or self-experiment, if that feels good to you. But it's also important to be able to figure out when it's time to get some lessons or even become a part of a bigger system of artisans.

Emulating a specific style or philosophy can be very attractive to some people. If you want to work in a well-established system of expression, such as classical Japanese painting or writing sonnets, you need to learn about the artistic and literary methods used in those pursuits. You can add your own touch or style, but your work will still become a part of a larger tradition. If this doesn't feel good to you, don't do it this way.

FINDING A TEACHER

Let's suppose you've decided that you would like to take some lessons. The next step involves finding the teacher who is right for you. To do this, you need to know about yourself: what your needs are, how you learn, and what you want to achieve. No one can tell you the answers to these questions—except yourself.

The ideal teacher for someone who is both ADD and creative is clearly someone who understands and respects both attributes. You need a teacher who is positive, who gives praise and positive feedback, and one who realizes the risk that people take when they open up creatively.

Be careful. Don't be misled by someone who tells you what you *should* learn or how you *should* learn. If someone believes in "no pain, no gain," run, don't walk, as far away from that teacher as you can—unless you enjoy pain for some reason. Otherwise, I promise you, there is no reason to put up with it.

Neither is there any reason to endure criticism. I mean *all* criticism. Yes, I've heard many people differentiate between constructive criticism and harmful criticism, but I would like to suggest another alternative. Rather than someone telling you what you are doing wrong, the teacher can first tell you what you are doing right, and what she wants.

Suppose you decided that you wanted to learn to improve your writing. Suppose your assignment was to write a story that could be submitted to a particular magazine. When your teacher looks at what you wrote, she might notice that your introduction is not strong enough to capture a publisher's or reader's attention. She'd like you to write a hard-hitting introduction. But instead of saying your introduction to the story is poor, or weak, or insufficient, she can say, "Let's talk about how to make the introduction to your story stronger." That becomes your lesson for the day.

Your teacher doesn't even need to point out what is inadequate about your work, but rather can show you the elements that make up a strong introduction. Then your assignment for your next lesson is to look back over the beginning of your story and strengthen it according to the teacher's guidelines and your own new skills.

She can also make a couple of suggestions about how to take what you've written and reword or reposition it so that it meets your goals better. Then she can ask you how you feel about the changes she has suggested—without automatically assuming that her suggestions are better than your work. She could ask, "Does this better reflect what you want?" If not, a good teacher will work with you until you *both* like and understand the changes. She will also tell you why she's suggesting what she's suggesting.

Asking Questions

If you're looking for a teacher who can guide you through some hands-on learning, find someone whose work you admire. This should be someone whose work you simply happen to like—not that you think you *should* like or because the person has a big reputation or because someone else likes him. The person you're considering does not necessarily have to be someone who is already officially a teacher. It could be someone who is very good at what he does but maybe has never before taken on a student.

How do you approach the person you'd like to study with? Be straightforward. Simply ask if he would take you on as a student. I'd suggest that you communicate through your choice of words the type of learning experience you are looking for—for example, how extensively you want to study, what your background is, and what you need or hope to get from the person.

Choose your words carefully. For example you might say, "Will you *show* me what to do," instead of "*tell* me what to do." Another phrase you could use is "walk me through it."

Then listen to his reply. If the person refers you to a book, he may not be the best person to teach someone who is ADD. If the person refers you to someone else's class, it may be his way of saying that he doesn't want to be a teacher but doesn't know how to say so directly.

If you are willing to clearly state your needs and desires, and if you are willing to listen carefully to your prospective teacher's response—putting aside what you would *like* to hear—you will eventually find the right mentor for you.

I used this method when I wanted to learn how to turn my poetry, monologues, and short stories into performing-arts pieces.

First, I went to the local theater and said that I'd like to learn about staging work and would be willing to help out behind the scenes to see how productions are put together. I explained that I thought that would be the best way for me to learn.

The director suggested that I audition for a part in the next production. My stomach churned, and I immediately knew this might not be the right place. I explained that I did not want to act or have to memorize lines. I was not interested in becoming an actress. He assumed that meant I had stage fright, which I don't. I love performing for an audience but only if it's an extemporaneous performance that doesn't require the memorization of lines.

After speaking with this man for a relatively short time, I realized he did not read me very well. But I made one more attempt to connect with him, asking if he'd look at some of my writings. I told him I wanted to know if he thought my work could be transferred to the stage. He took my pieces and said he would look at them. After a month, I called him to ask if he'd read my work. He said he had been too busy. By the end of the second month, I simply asked for them back. I realized that this person was not going to be the teacher for me.

Next, I went to a community theater production in a nearby town. After enjoying the performance, I sought out the director. I told him the same thing: I'd like to learn about theater production and I learn best by doing rather than by reading or by hearing about what to do. The director talked to me for some time and told me I could come and watch the construction of the children's production that was just going into rehearsal.

I ended up as a props manager and learned a lot. I did the same for a second production. But I also discovered that I was so busy with the production, there was no time to work on my writing with anyone. I had to remember that my ultimate goal was to work on my writing, to turn it into a format that could be performed.

So I continued to talk about my interests with people I met. Through that sharing and networking, I found that the Austin poetry scene provided just the opportunity I had been looking for. Some of the women poets decided to join forces to create a performing-arts evening. Several of them knew of my interest and asked me to come to a planning meeting, which I was excited to do.

I took part in our first performance a few months ago. I had my very own eight-minute segment with six of my poems set to music, and dancers expressing a physical picture of the poems.

Our group continued to work together, and my new goal became the development of enough material so that I could put on a whole show myself. But, knowing that I needed more experience in order to be able to do that, I kept looking for people I could learn from.

Fortuitously, I met a man at a party who had worked extensively in theater, and I asked him to join a writer's group at my home. This informal, noncritical, supportive group provides a place where several of us brainstorm and draw encouragement from like-minded people.

I asked the group as a whole how they thought I could take two poems, two monologues, and a short story and weave them into a cohesive production. The man I had recently met immediately saw one angle that I'd never thought of, and he asked for copies of the works in question. I could see his mind working, strategizing how to weave the pieces together. I gave him the copies of my work the next day. And I'm looking forward to learning from his ideas.

The point is that when you have a desire to learn something, you must keep trying to find the teacher you need. Just don't quit. You may be fortunate and find *the* teacher right away. Then again, you may put together pieces of teachers, like I've done so far. Either way, just keep going!

TAKE CHARGE OF THE SITUATION

Remember that, as a student, you are a consumer. The product you're buying is the lesson you're taking. If the lesson doesn't meet your needs or your requirements, you need to speak up.

I'm not saying that's always an easy thing to do. I understand that many people with ADD have feelings of insecurity and low self-esteem brought on by years of difficulties with the standard educational system, difficulties that can lead them to believe that something is wrong with them—when the problem actually lies in the lack of fit between their learning methods and the system's teaching methods.

Feeling insecure or having low self-esteem can cause you to censor what you say and cause you to not speak up for yourself. But your creative self needs you to speak up so you can get what you need from your teacher.

Be as clear as you can when you are stating your needs to your prospective teacher. Initially, however, you might not be sure exactly what you are looking for. In that case, you might want to say, "All I know is that I want to learn to do something with the stage. I don't know exactly what that is, but I will figure it out as I get involved, and I'll let you know." Then ask if that's okay with the teacher. Your job, then, is to keep your teacher abreast of what you want, as you discover it for yourself.

As you continue with the learning process, you will develop a deeper understanding of your needs in relation to the subject you're studying. As your needs and directions change, be sure to share that information with your teacher. When we were children, we were always told to finish anything we started. But as adults, we have the power to make changes if we don't like the direction we've been taking. It's important to always remember that.

Let's say you are learning to do desktop publishing and have learned the basics to design a pamphlet or set up a booklet. Sure, there is a lot more you can learn about desktop publishing, but you feel that what you've learned so far is adequate to meet your needs for now. But maybe you really have a desire to explore computer animation instead, because you feel that your creative goals will better be met that way. So you change software and begin to learn about animation. After a bit you may discover that your interest again turns in another direction. Don't automatically assume that this pattern means you *never* finish things or that you are distractible. It's just possible that what you've just learned—either from desktop publishing or computer animation—will be applied in whatever new area you decide to study next.

Many creative people do this. They take one skill from here, a bit from there and something else from another arena. Then they put together a combination of skills or talents in a creative way and come up with something new. After all, isn't that what creativity is all about?

When you come to a difference of opinion with your teacher, don't always assume that you are wrong, and the teacher is right. Of course, don't *blame* the teacher either. Instead, try to be constructive in your conversations with your teacher. Make suggestions that you think might work better for you. For example, you can say, "I don't understand what you are telling me to do. I don't know if it's my understanding or the way you're saying it, but can you show me a different way, or tell me a different way?"

If your teacher suggests that you undertake something that doesn't feel right or that makes you very uncomfortable, say so. Suggest that you go in another direction for now. Maybe you'll come back to the skipped lesson later when you are ready for it, or maybe that lesson is just not meant to be a part of your learning experience. Only time will tell.

When I was learning to throw pots back in the sixties, one of the things I had to learn was how to make a glaze. I made a few that were great. But I wasn't able to keep track of the chemicals I'd put into them, so I could never replicate them. I tried to keep track of the chemicals, just like I tried to pass qualitative analysis in college. But both are totally beyond my capability, because I manage to make new mistakes or repeat old mistakes every time I try for a particular outcome.

I decided that glazing was just too much work for me. I also didn't much care for the commercial premade glazes that were on the market. So I concentrated on making unglazed pottery and sculpture that emphasized the use of different clays and carving techniques. I had a wonderful time. I found that my productions reflected the earthiness that has come to symbolize my true nature. In some strange way my inability to replicate glazes consistently opened the door to my finding a technique that suited me very well. I very much liked the end result. But if I had not given myself the freedom to give up on glazing and go in a new direction, I would never have discovered a technique that fit me so well.

Obviously, my viewpoint means that you would be wise to refrain from signing up for a long-term series of classes. A few weeks at a time is a good-size commitment. I do understand that teachers need to make a living, but I also know that a flexible teacher who is there to meet students' needs understands that learning situations are not static. That's the kind of teacher you need to find. The students of flexible teachers return regularly when they're ready for a next step. They also refer a lot of other students to their teacher. In the long run, a flexible teacher will build a better business.

If you find that you have overcommitted, either moneywise, timewise, or commitmentwise, the best thing to do is to talk to your teacher about it. You can say, "When I signed up with you, I did not realize the direction my interests would take me. I apologize for any inconvenience I may be causing you, but I need a refund or I need to cut back my hours." And you can say, "I want to thank you for the time you've spent with me. You've helped get me ready for the next step I want to take."

A really good teacher knows when the student is ready to move on to study with someone who has different skills than he possesses. After all, a teacher can only carry a student as far as that teacher has gone and as far as the student is interested in going.

If you keep the lines of communication open between you and your teacher, you won't end up with any surprises. Remember, you are the one who is ultimately responsible for building a learning program that fits you.

No one else can do that without input from you.

Recognizing the True Teaching-Learning Process

How can you recognize when you've found the right teacher? How do you know when the learning process is just what it should be for you, as an adult? Here are some guidelines.

When things are going right, you will feel free to make mistakes.

You will not feel judged on your production.

You won't be graded on your work.

You will come away from lessons with hope and enthusiasm for your work.

You will feel that you are making progress most of the time.

Your teacher won't enter you into competitions. Competitions are not constructive to openness and learning until the very latest stages of your learning.

You will be provided with opportunities to showcase your work *if you desire*, but *only* if you desire.

You will be given encouragement because your work is seen as valuable.

You will receive positive feedback because your teacher sees value and quality in your work and can point these out to you.

You will learn something new on a regular basis.

You will feel that you and your teachers are partners in education—not that your teacher is more important in the relationship and you are less important.

In a true teacher-learner relationship, both parties grow and learn.

You deserve this kind of treatment when you are a student. Be sure that you get it.

My Music Lessons

Like many people who are ADD and creative, I have faced a lot of struggles in finding a teacher I can really learn from. Those struggles have made me acutely aware of what can go wrong in this educational process. But things can also go right. I know that now, because I have found a music composition teacher who emulates the attributes that I've listed above. I've learned how wonderful a good student-teacher relationship can be.

I would like to share my personal learning experience as an example that may touch familiar chords in you—my experiences with music.

My story begins as a very young child. I vaguely recall taking piano lessons when I was four or five. I had a great desire to do well, but I remember always feeling that I wasn't doing well enough. I lived in fear—fear of failure. Now I realize that a lot of my problem was the fact that I wasn't able to sit still long enough to practice much. At the time, of course, I had no idea what the problem was.

No one beat me. I don't remember my teacher really criticizing me. But somehow I sensed that I didn't produce what I could have if I had practiced more.

The lessons also seemed boring and the music very different from the lively music I liked to listen to. Perhaps I just couldn't imagine how I would get from the music I could produce at my level of skill to the music I liked to listen to. Since no one knew how I felt, no one told me that my problem was a common one for children of my age, children who need to be reassured that their musical skills will improve over time and that the music they will make will be more to their liking.

My piano lessons made me feel boxed in. They were never a creative experience for me. Yet I loved music and wanted to be involved with it. As a teen I played my piano at home for many hours on my own, reading the music that was handed down to me. I played, but I didn't practice. Over time I became modestly capable, though I never played for anyone else.

In fifth through twelfth grades, I studied the saxophone—prompted by my dad. This was not my instrument of choice, and again I didn't practice much, though I did spend a lot of time feeling guilty because I wasn't practicing. I did okay with the saxophone. But, again, I definitely was not performing at a level that would reflect my real love for music.

When I was a teenager, a small group of us got together to form a band. I think we had a piano, clarinet, drums, and my saxophone. There may have been a bass player, too. We met quite a bit for a while, but none of us really knew what we were doing. I recall transposing a little music, but I didn't know how to arrange music, nor did the others. And none of us knew how to improvise. Basically we had a lot of interest in music but no guidance or innate skill to have a musical jam session.

Along the way I also had some experience in conducting a small school band. I loved doing that. However, since I have a poor sense of tone, I faced limitations in working with so many instruments at one time. Besides, girls didn't go into professions such as conducting.

But I did earn a scholarship to college to play in the band. I even considered music as a career. But I knew there were too many pieces missing in my sense of music for that to be a wise choice. I had no idea what I'd do with such a degree. I didn't have *the feel* of music then. I also never exercised the scholarship. I became fearful that I wouldn't be able to keep up and withdrew before the first practice. I felt someone had made a mistake giving it to me in the first place.

In retrospect I knew so little about the music world, it's really remarkable that I even considered it for a vocation. But I did have a deep desire to create music.

After high school my life went a different direction that did not involved music. My piano was sold, and I shut the door on music in my life. I rarely even listened to it. When I did, I'd often start to cry. I would hear classics that made my heart soar. Or I would hear contemporary tunes that made my feet want to dance. But I married a nondancer, and I felt awful listening to music that made me want to dance when I couldn't.

Later, when I was single again, I recall wanting very much to dance, but I couldn't find a partner to dance with. I agonized over this lack, prayed about it, and tried a few times to just show up where people were dancing. But the experience was less than positive, so I gave up on that. I didn't know then about the dance opportunities I enjoy now—authentic dance, expressive dance, and movement where no partner is needed.

I had also wanted to play an organ for years because I like the sustained nature of the tones. So a few years ago, I bought one and excitedly sat down to see what I could do. I signed up for weekly lessons. Two things became immediately clear to me. First, I really didn't want to learn to play the organ in any formal way. I liked being able to use it to make a lot of sound easily, but I wasn't interested in studying it to achieve technical proficiency. Second, though I would often play for an hour or two in the evening for my own amusement, I didn't want to practice as an adult any more than I did as a kid.

I told my teacher of my awareness and that I would like to learn to play with flexibility and freedom. He began to teach me about making chords that would go with a melody. He explained a little about music theory—fifths, fourths, intervals, and I chords, II chords, IV chords, and so forth, in different keys. My head started to swim. I felt nauseous, and I wanted to cry.

When I went home that day, I sat down and wrote a story. I'm going to share that story with you now because I think it will help you understand the frustrations that an ill-fitting "learning" experience brings to someone with ADD and creativity. Reading about the fact the someone with ADD and creativity needs a certain type of teacher is one thing. Feeling the intensity of that need is something else again.

Let the Music Begin

A little girl sits upright on a piano bench. Her feet reach the pedals because she is encased in the body of a grown woman; one accomplished in her own right, successful by most people's standards, often sought for her skills.

The child feels afraid but she dares not tell anyone. So she holds her breath. The woman bites her lip, fearful that she'll burst out crying, sobbing the pain she feels inside.

The woman's mind dances from thought to thought, aware of feelings that demand action on her part so they can come under her control. She knows they are not in response to her teacher. He is kind, reserved, not the least bit threatening. But she can't deny the hesitation her adult legs endured as they moved toward the studio. And her heart felt tugged, pulled into elongated form, reaching for the spot in the center of her solar plexus where all her deepest feelings lie in wait to be comforted and protected.

On this day the child within her needs protection more than comfort. The woman knows her child is close to panic, because she has to stop breathing momentarily to keep control. The pressure to run, scream, hide her eyes behind her hands can only come from one so young—maybe five.

"All right, it's time to deal with this," she whispers to the child.

"I have something I need to let you know," the woman tells the teacher. "I'm having trouble performing the pieces I've been practicing this week. I guess I'm afraid I'll make a mistake."

Comfortingly, he responds with reassurances about mistakes.

But somehow that doesn't feel entirely right to the woman. It's not quite the feeling. It's not a mistake that she fears. Though that would be a logical assumption. The idea that making mistakes is a problem is more of a thought than a feeling. And it doesn't even hurt to think it. No, it's not the fear of making a mistake that is causing the trouble today.

Offering this conclusion to the teacher, she continues to focus her attention to a place in her chest where her heart and her child's merge, leaking their vital fluid into the reservoir of her midsection so that tension is tautly strung from her throat to just above her navel. As it tightens, relief threatens to come from the release of tears. "No!" she says to herself and bites her lip hard again.

The woman's brain scans the situation and continues to listen to the teacher. She shares her awareness of her five-year-old with him and in return hears the empathy that comes from many years of teaching children as well as adults. But that doesn't do the trick. The learning opportunity has not yielded to understanding yet.

Silently she murmurs to her child, "Hang in there, sweet one. I'll not leave you. I never do. We'll find the core of this issue and you, I, and it will heal."

"You know," she says to the teacher, "I can talk before thousands of people and it doesn't bother me. The words just come. Others ask how I do it, but I don't know. It's just automatic, easy, and always has been. But playing the pieces isn't easy. It's not automatic . . ."

It's then that the woman remembers how it had been in school trying to read—the same way, hard. No, reading wasn't just hard, it was impossible. But there is something else. She knew she was never afraid of hard work, but work so difficult that it made no sense was too much to endure. That's a different feeling, and she is experiencing it now. Right now! It's helplessness.

There it is! The woman feels the pain. The child lives the pain.

It's a feeling of being totally helpless to do anything about learning what she wants to learn and *knows* she can understand. She tried hard to practice, and still she did not retain the lessons. She didn't know what to do.

And now an old physical feeling makes its way into her consciousness. It's located in her head. She feels the right side of her head throbbing, stretching, trying to encapsulate the information. The left side of her mind is dark and blank. She can't feel anything beyond its edges. She sees the right side speaking, reacting spontaneously, creating. The left remains quiet, empty.

The pain surges deep within, engulfing the child who was so bright, creative, and skillful and, yet, so unable to learn her lessons. The woman's eyes again reflect the depth of her little one's helplessness. "Breathe," she says, "breathe, child."

That's it! All the remembered times of not being able to do what she wanted to do: to think right, produce right, even feel right. The death of her learning brain, the greatest terror she can imagine, already occurred, marring her joy for more than half a century. And today she revisits the graveside, her child in hand.

This doesn't really have to do with anyone else. It's a loss experienced by her and her child, and they'll grieve together. Whether or not the mastery of music lessons is achieved takes a back seat to the release of pent up memories etched in the archives of personal history. The healing of a psyche and soul are at stake, and that will be honored. Perhaps then, sweet music can be played from the hands, mind, and heart of a child freed within the body of the woman she's become.

And so it is!

The week after I wrote this story, I let my music teacher read it. What a risk—at least that's how it felt to me. He opened his eyes wide and thanked me. He instructed me to let him know if he went too fast. In retrospect I know he didn't really understand what was happening to me. Neither did I, really. But he was kind, and I knew he didn't intend to hurt me or even make things difficult for me. I did learn to manage some chords in a few keys, but not by *learning* the theory. I just gradually began to be able to use them. That was fun.

But the lessons themselves caused at least as much frustration as pleasure. Every time he began to explain music theory, I gasped for breath, cried inside and wanted to run. I found myself wondering what my inner desire to create music was really all about.

Shortly after I asked myself that question, I came across a poem I'd written called "How to Make a Rainbow." After rereading it, I felt I wanted to put it to music. I could envision it being danced on a stage with the narration of the poem set to music. As I felt each line of the poem, I felt the feeling the words conveyed. Then I saw designs in my mind that expressed those feelings, and I drew the designs. Then I felt how these designs, line by line, would become music—for I've always seen pictures when I hear music. The resulting musical phrases created feelings that replicated the original feelings of the poetry. It is as if I first saw pictures of the feelings and then could create music to replicate the same feelings.

Later I sat down at the organ, looked at the designs I'd drawn, and created the musical phrases that made me feel the same way the pictures made me feel. This is how I wrote the music for the whole poem—in one sitting. I really can't remember *thinking* about any of it. It just wrote itself. When I finished, I felt satisfied, thrilled, and complete.

At my next lesson I told my teacher that I wanted to learn to compose. Then I showed him the "Rainbow" piece. Although he was willing to shift gears with me to focus on writing music, that meant more music theory. Sometimes I would understand what he was saying in class, but as soon as I had arrived home I'd forgotten it all. Other times, I didn't even understand what he was saying as he said it. No matter how hard I tried, I just couldn't get it.

At about that time I saw a television show about composers. In the show the statement was made that if you can't structure and control your music according to the discipline of music theory, you aren't writing good music. I instantly became enraged at what I felt was the arrogance of the comment. But when I looked closer at my feelings, I found, under the anger, the heartbreaking feelings of inadequacy. I desperately wanted to learn how to structure and control my music. But I just couldn't seem to do it.

I kept at my music lessons, but it eventually became apparent that I was not going to be able to learn to write music by learning music theory. My teacher and

How to Make a Rainbow

Massage emotion,
The energies of which
Were never before vibrated,
Sliding by each other
As Sweetness.

> *Then fear*
> *Slashes,*
> *In between.*

Torid play,
Touches the ices of terror.
Tension,

> *Long since made rigid by hurt.*

> *Windswept*
> *By deliberateness,*
> *The touch*

Releases a mini-amp of charge,

Thread by thread,

Cord next to chord,

Sheathed between layers of color.

I were both becoming frustrated by the situation. I wanted to quit my lessons, but I was afraid that if I did, I'd never be able to fulfill my dream of composing.

I did the only thing I know to do when I don't know what to do. I prayed. I know that prayer is a deeply personal topic and that it might or might not apply to your life. For myself, I have to be honest with you. I couldn't imagine how in the world I could learn to write music if I couldn't learn music theory. But I have a faith that allows for unlimited potential, and I simply released my desire to a power greater than mine.

Within a couple of days I found myself thinking about a young man whom I'd met a few months earlier, a musician who had encouraged me after I told him what I was doing with my music. I picked up the phone and asked him if he would be willing to try to teach me how to write music. He said yes. He told me to bring the music I'd written, and we'd start there.

From my first lesson with Jerell, I knew I was talking to someone who spoke my language. Jerell understood and respected what I did and did not need to teach theory. We communicated about feelings, and I told him how much I desired to turn my writing into music. I played a piece I'd started composing, a piece that was based on some of my writing. But I was stuck on it and couldn't seem to get the direction to continue or finish it. He asked me some questions about the sense and tone that I wanted to create. I found myself talking with my hands, drawing the pictures of the feelings in the air. I told him how I wanted the music to follow those same lines.

I told him that I wasn't sure exactly what it was I was writing. He thought about it and responded it was sort of like a Greek drama or a musical drama. Opera would be too formal a word, but I liked the term "musical drama," so that's what I called it. I was excited. My potential creation had a name, and it was beginning to take on a form of its own—which meant that I would be able to connect with it.

At the next lesson he showed me a symphony that he'd written and explained how he'd outlined the "musical characters" by composing musical phrases that would repeat throughout the symphony. Now that was something I could instantly understand. I could also get a handle on the individual "characters" of my piece in the same way.

I had hope.

At that point an opportunity presented itself for me to showcase six of my poems, including the one that I'd written the music for, "How to Make a Rainbow." Jerell agreed to write the music for the other five poems and arranged "Rainbow."

A week later Jerell presented me with sketches of the music he was outlining for the poems. He also described them with his hands. I instantly saw that he'd captured the tone of the poems. Delighted, I said, "I can understand what you are planning to do. I love it. How have you managed to communicate so clearly to me?"

His response made me laugh and cry at the same time. "I joined your system," he said. "I drew you pictures that you could read." My mind shouted with joy, "He understands. And *I* understand in a way I've never before been able to." It fits!

I don't know where all of this is going to take me. I don't even know now whether or how much I need to continue to write music. But I do know that I understand the process and that music is becoming integrated into everything I do.

I find it interesting that I didn't really say much to Jerell about my being ADD when we started working together. We talked a little about how people learn, and he shared how he seems to learn. He's what I call a "bridge person." He has some wiring in my camp and some in the linear camp. He can build bridges between the two camps, and he doesn't make judgments about one or the other. He utilizes skills from both and acknowledges both equally.

Now we talk a lot about ADD because we've both become very interested in how people learn. I teach him and he teaches me. I suspect we'll come out of this student-teacher relationship with a lot more understanding about how people learn than we intended when I first called him.

When I look at the list of the characteristics that make a good teacher-learner relationship, I realize Jerell has all the "good teacher" attributes. The man is a natural, gifted teacher as well as a fine musician and talented composer. I am fortunate to have found him.

Now I know that my inability to learn was not just because of me but it was a matter of not having found my fit, the one I needed before I could release my ability. I know there are no bad guys in this scenario, but I also know how important it is to find a teacher with whom you're compatible.

Don't give up. Keep looking for the teacher who is right for you. You, too, will find the gem at the end of the rainbow. You deserve it.

chapter ten

Overcoming Practical Problems

S A TWENTY-ONE-YEAR-OLD college student Jackson designed a waste treatment program as part of a class assignment. His instructor not only marked the project with an A but told Jackson he thought the program had real potential for commercial use. Jackson felt excited and motivated to go out into the world and make a difference. Up until then he had struggled to get through school, even though he felt smart. His difficulty with learning had never quite made sense to him. But his teacher's feedback gave him confidence.

Two years after his instructor's suggestion Jackson had made little progress. At first he spent many hours continuing to develop the plans. He checked into governmental regulations but never got very far in trying to figure out how to meet them. He wanted to start his own business but dealing with financial plans, budgets and paperwork proved to be much more difficult for him than designing the prototypical plant. Then Jackson thought about trying to sell his idea to an already established company, but he didn't really know how to go about that either.

Jackson did know how to make friends, but he didn't know how to network to achieve business goals. He tended to make decisions about people based on how much he liked them rather than on their skills. He vacillated between fearing he'd be cheated and trying to give his ideas and plans away for the betterment of the community. At the end of two years, Jackson was completely confused and didn't know where to turn. Financially, he'd made it through somehow, but now he had to make a living full time.

So Jackson turned to landscape work. He started his own business doing what he liked to do—designing commercial and residential outdoor areas. He figured it ought to be simple enough to bid a job and do the work himself. However, Jackson forgot about the paperwork, taxes, collections, timely ordering of supplies, and a multitude of other details. He also forgot about proper planning. Jackson would commit to creative projects he really wanted to do before checking his schedule and often wouldn't be able to follow through. Consequently, his business never ran smoothly. He became frustrated, and his temper got out of control.

Jackson's impulsivity, temper, and lack of organizational skills caught up with him before too long. He found himself in debt, in trouble with the IRS, and missing his truck—an essential for work—because he'd fallen too far behind in his payments.

Jackson finally gave up his business and took a job for another contractor, but that didn't last long either. Jackson wanted to be creative in everything he did, but his boss just wanted to get the job done. The day he was let go, his boss told him, "Jackson, I can't use you. Yes, your work is beautiful. But I can't afford to pay you for that quality of work. I told you two weeks ago that you need to get the jobs done the way I tell you and quit improvising. But your work is still coming in late. I have to let you go. You need to be on your own."

Chances are, you can relate to at least some of Jackson's difficulties. Those of us who are ADD and creative share some common issues that can make it difficult for us to accomplish what we would really like to do. In this chapter we'll take a look at those issues and some solutions.

The end goal is to allow you to enjoy your creativity and be successful utilizing it—never to try to avoid the issues by changing you into a noncreative, non-ADD person. I want you to be yourself *and* be successful and happy.

SELF-DISCIPLINE

If you are ADD, you probably have some difficulty with self-discipline. But have you ever considered why that might be the case? The reason for your difficulty is that you have been asked to do things that don't fit—for as long as you can remember. Ordinarily, people don't develop self-discipline for something that doesn't fit. That's because when someone is asked to do something he isn't comfortable doing, he usually needs someone outside of himself to constantly prod and push him to continue. That's no way to develop *self*-discipline

The word self is present in self-discipline for a reason. It means that you hold the power within yourself to accomplish a task. It means you take the responsibility in your own hands to reach a goal. To do that, you have to be familiar with that place inside yourself that is in control of getting things done. But that part will never develop if you're constantly being forced to do things that don't fit.

Once that inner piece is in place, then you can use it to accomplish whatever you want—and even some things that you don't much want. You will use it to *be disciplined*.

GETTING STARTED

Have you ever had twenty-five ideas jumping around in your head all at one time? Have you ever thought about four or five wonderfully exciting creative projects all at the same time, any one of which seemed like a good bet for making money? If you are ADD, the answer is probably, "Sure."

So where do you start? Chances are you enthusiastically start one—often the one that is closest at hand—and run with it until you hit your first roadblock or delay. Then you start the next one and run with it until it hits a snag, and so forth. Before you know it, you've got several projects going at once.

I do realize that some people who are ADD can do more than one thing at a time effectively. But if you're trying to keep track of more than three or four projects at once, chances are you've bitten off more than you or anyone can chew.

Be honest, now. I don't want you losing out or cheating yourself out of success. Let's look at what goes on in your mind.

When you first begin a project, you probably feel excitement. Sound familiar? Then all too quickly, does confusion take over, followed by panic that you will *never accomplish anything substantial?*

People who are ADD and creative have no problem coming up with ideas for projects. But, in contrast, planning and organizing those projects is usually painful, out of our grasp, and anxiety-producing. That's just the way our ADD brains are wired. We do the creative stuff easily. Handling the myriad details is a totally different matter.

Another reason why you may have such a hard time choosing one project and following through on it stems from your experience with the many, many uncompleted projects strewn around you. Surrounded by a historical graveyard of uncompleted tasks, you are probably quite anxious about your ability to achieve success. So grabbing three projects to work on at a time is like having two projects for insurance purposes when the first one doesn't get completed. Unfortunately, however, the second and third ones not only make an easy out

173

when you hit a roadblock with the first project, but are probably also a distraction, disrupting your work on the first.

I want to share some tips with you that I've learned because I want you to know the joy of a completed project. You can accomplish anything you want—it just takes time, flexibility, and stick-to-itiveness. That doesn't mean that you will necessarily complete the project in one sitting or before you do anything else, but it does mean that you give it everything you've got. It means that if you decide to set it aside, you know where you put it and how to get back to it. For example, suppose you were repairing cars. If you were waiting on a part to come in for one car, you would set that one aside and start working on another. When the part came in for the first car, you would go back to work on that.

Whether your project is car repair or cleaning your room, you can accomplish the project. As soon as the needed piece of information or aspect of the project comes to you—whether that's a car part, a note you wrote to yourself that you misplaced, or a phone call you've been waiting for—you can retrieve the original project that takes priority over the one you started while you were waiting.

So how do you decide where to start? When you are choosing which project to begin first, I'd strongly suggest you choose something that is small and simple and something that you really want to do. At the beginning don't worry about how you're going to accomplish the larger, more complicated project down the road. Just start with something small and simple. That way you'll quickly have a successful experience.

For example, let's say you want to learn to knit or crochet. Instead of starting on a quilt for a king-sized bed, start with the cover for a small pillow or a tiny scarf. You could even start with a small kit to get the hang of the skills involved before jumping off and buying a lot of materials.

If your creativity is offended by the idea of using a kit, you might change the colors suggested in it, or create your own design. Doing the work still builds your skills. Maybe you decide to not finish the kit because you have learned what you are doing, and you feel ready to go on to a project that excites you. In that case purposely set the kit aside. You might give it to a senior center or a friend so it doesn't go to waste.

It's important to be clear in your mind that you aren't quitting or giving up on that first project. It's not that you couldn't finish it. It's that you've purposely chosen not to because you've gained what you wanted from it—learning the steps of a new skill. Remind yourself that you are in charge of the choices you are making.

Next, be sure to choose a project that excites you. Don't do something just because someone else tells you to, including me. If you choose a project because you are excited about it, your heightened motivation will provide you with fuel for a while to keep the project going. It may not be enough to carry you through to the end, but it can give you a good start. As you move through the project, you can purposely boost your motivation level with breaks, cheerleading from a friend or colleague, or the promise of reward at the end.

Whatever project you pick, I would suggest picking one and only one. I know how hard that is. But bite the bullet and know that it doesn't matter which one you begin with. Good projects never get lost. Mediocre and bad projects fall by the wayside, but you don't really need them anyway. You will have enough *great* projects that come to you continuously that you do not need to worry about your creativity drying up.

Simply pick one. You can meet with success no matter which one you pick. Linear thinkers strategize to figure out which one is best. They collect data to figure out which one will yield the best bottom line or outcome. But there is little point in your trying to use this method. What usually happens for ADD/creative thinkers is that they get so bogged down in making a business plan or trying to figure the way linear thinkers do, that they don't ever get to the project.

Just pick one. Yes, the one you like best. Or the one that touches your heart most deeply. Maybe it will be the one that's hung around in your mind the longest. As an ADD/creative thinker, you'll probably end up making your choice by using your feelings, not a linear strategy.

Once you've chosen which project to begin, be prepared for criticism from friends or family who are linear thinkers. They will probably tell you that you didn't go about choosing your project the right way. Even many nonlinear thinkers who have been brainwashed into believing that you have to go through all kinds of mental gymnastics to accomplish a project will be critical of your approach.

But I'm telling you to *use your feelings*. They won't lie for you. You have as great a chance of success as the non feelings decision makers. Besides, the other method won't work for you because your brain is wired in a different way.

What I'm telling you fits the way your brain is wired. Your feelings *will* work for you. Trust me.

DECIDING ON YOUR AGENDA

Once you have a creative project in mind, you need to decide what you want to get out of the project. You might not automatically think about doing this. But it is very important. If you don't purposely sit down and make that decision, you set yourself up to get lost and confused and you will tend to work inefficiently.

Ask yourself these questions: Do I want to turn my project into a product that can be sold? Is it just for my own amusement? Do I want to do the project to learn something?

Most people with ADD do not automatically differentiate between these goals due to our lack of clear boundaries. Since we think globally, goals don't jump out at us. So this is an opportunity to use your thinking mind to clarify your goals.

Once you've made your selection, you can move onto the next step and clearly define your first tangible plans and the process needed to meet your goal.

First Steps

There is no one right way to start a project. I prefer to get someone to help me construct an outline because that keeps me on track and assures completion. I like to get things done, but I have difficulty outlining projects—planning out the order in which the steps should be done. I can't decide what needs to go first, then second. By the time I reach step ten or eleven, I'm lost. I end up with about five tracks that I need to take care of all at once. Then I become frustrated.

My solution—which I first learned while writing books and have since applied to other types of projects—has been to team with people who are wired differently than me. Sometimes I hire someone to work for me, sometimes I make trades or partner with the person and sometimes I accept favors. But whatever arrangements are made, I respect the skills that the more linear-minded person brings to the table. I know that having brought those skills to my project from an outside source, I can get on with what I do so well, which is to create.

I also don't necessarily start at what would seem to be the logical beginning of a project. There is nothing wrong with starting midstream or at the end of a creation and working sideways or backwards. What you need to do is listen to the promptings of the creative part of yourself. You may decide to start wherever your attention falls. Go for it! You are the creative one and you know better than anyone else how to do your creating.

Chances are you're hearing the voice that says, "You have to start at the beginning and have a structure and do things sequentially or you will have a lot of repair work to do later." I hear that voice, too. My response is, "Maybe yes, maybe no."

When we have taken a linear approach to creative work, many of us who are ADD have failed to achieve the outcomes we wanted. When that happens, the assumption is that if you had just been better organized, you would not have had so much trouble. But I have begun to think that maybe the failure is more the result of not using our own way of proceeding: Failing to listen to our feelings and follow what we feel inside. The more I encourage creative ADD people to do this, the more successful they become—even though they may not be able to explain exactly how they got their results to someone who doesn't have faith in their own feelings or understand the creative process.

When I do creative art and creative writing, I do not use outlines. I listen; I shift into a relaxed frame of mind and body and wait for a cue. That cue might be a picture, something I notice in my environment, or a sound or word in my mind. One of these cues invariably gets the process started. Then I don't have a conscious thought until the piece is finished. If I am working on a larger creative piece, I divide it into segments and apply the same process to each segment.

This is a very different kind of work from writing a self-help book about ADD. There is a place for both types of projects, and I understand each. They are different projects with different types of outcomes, and they require different methods of work.

I am not "disordered" because I can't make a linear outline any more than a linear thinker is "disordered" because he can't create a poem without a plan or outline formulated ahead of time.

We are just different from one another.

Sticking with It

The general consensus is that people with ADD are reactive and pulled off track by what's going on around them. But my view is slightly different. What I see is that the worse the fit is between the person doing the project and the structure of the project, the more the person will be pulled off track by whatever is going on around her or him.

For example, if someone with ADD is doing an art project that is very free and creative and he is very much into it, he would probably not be pulled off track by anything. But if this same person is forced to sit in a school desk for three straight hours and answer final-exam questions by filling in dots on an answer sheet, chances are his is going to be constantly distracted and pulled off track by any little thing going on in the room—whether or not he knows the material.

But think about it in reverse. A linear person might be able to zip through three hours of that final exam. But she might feel very uncomfortable and unable to concentrate if she were handed a paintbrush in an art class and asked to paint a picture of "cold." Would that linear thinker be labeled disordered? I think not.

The better the fit, the more you will be able to accomplish any goal you set for yourself and stick with it. That's true no matter what your brain wiring happens to be.

All people who are ADD are not wired identically, nor do they respond the same way when doing a project. You may hyper-focus, in which case you may wish to stay with the project from beginning to end. There's nothing wrong with that—as long as you realize that you do need rest and relaxation along the way so you don't burn out, abuse your body and mind, or offend others.

Maybe you prefer to work for a short period of time and then take a break, which can be looked at as a reward, then work again, then take a break, and so on. There's nothing wrong with this pattern, either. You just have to be sure that short breaks don't become extended breaks.

For example, I'll always remember the man who rewarded himself for doing work he didn't like by reading a chapter of a book. The chapters were about twenty pages long and served the purpose well. However, one day, as he was finishing his break he realized he'd been reading for over an hour. It turns out that the chapter he read was seventy pages long. From then on he changed his reward to reading twenty pages regardless of whether it was a chapter or not.

There's another element to sticking with a project, one that's possibly more important than finding a work schedule that fits you well. You need to look at what you believe about yourself. Do you *expect* that you will fail? That's the best way to set yourself up to not finish what you start.

I realize you may have a long history of failing. But think about what you were trying to do. Weren't you often attempting something that really didn't fit you? If so, your failure to finish your project only proves that you got off track because you were trying to do something that doesn't fit you. It does not prove that you will get off track from doing something that *does* fit you.

Take a minute to think about that again. Any past failures have nothing to do with your chances of future success if you undertake a project that fits you properly. That is the truth, and you need to believe in it.

Start today with a new attitude, committed to doing only projects that you truly want to do. As you proceed, be aware of fears that well up inside of you. Listen for dialogue in your mind that questions your adequacy and ability to do the job successfully.

You'll find that as soon as your mental voice says, "You're not doing a good enough job for this to succeed," you will immediately get distracted by something, anything, that gets you away from the awful feeling of being a failure again. Or, if you notice that someone else is doing something similar and you feel sure that your product won't be as good—after all, it never was in the past—you will tend to lose your motivation and easily become distracted.

Finally, you need to become aware of when you have reached a stage in a project that is very difficult for you to do. For example, Shawn was a college student who loved creating projects and papers for school. He liked reading about the subject he'd picked and thoroughly enjoyed thinking about the implications of what he was reading. But when it came to organizing his material so that he could write the paper, Shawn got off track. Suddenly he would become hungry, need a drink of water, remember an errand that absolutely had to be done at that exact moment, hear the fan rattling and decide it needed to be oiled, think of another paper he had to write, notice notes from his class laying by his work table, and so on. He would become distracted by absolutely anything and everything in his environment or in his mind.

The problem for Shawn was that he didn't know how to organize his materials—neither did he know how to get past that roadblock. When he got stuck at that point in the process, he became easily distracted. Shawn didn't realize why he was getting off track and why he was failing to stick with the assigned goal. He figured it was just his ADD kicking in. Others, to be sure, thought of him as not having stick-to-itiveness. They advised Shawn to take medication so he could concentrate. The whole point was missed.

In order to successfully complete projects, you must become aware of the situations that set you up to be easily distracted. Check your feelings and your thinking. When you become distracted, ask yourself if you are at a "stuck" part of a project. Ask yourself if you want to proceed but just aren't sure how to get past your roadblock. Be as clear with yourself when you *can't* do something as you are when you *can*.

Realize, too, that there is nothing wrong with not knowing how to do whatever you are struggling with. No one does everything well—I don't, the college professor doesn't, and the artist who's won ten awards for her work doesn't. Every one of us has strengths and weaknesses. It's identifying your own strengths and weaknesses that can put you ahead of the game. That's when you can compensate for your weaknesses and utilize your strengths to their fullest.

Another View on Being Self-Disciplined

What you have been reading about has to do with the problems faced by many people who are ADD and who have had trouble developing self-discipline. But there are some of us who present a different picture.

Some people with ADD develop a tremendous, almost destructive, amount of self-discipline from the time they are very young. They have a fierce drive to work in order to prove that they can be just like everyone else. This becomes such a way of life for some people with ADD that even when they don't know how to do something, they pretend to work at it. They work so hard that they often lose part of themselves in the process.

This kind of work ethic, lauded by our culture, comes as a response to feeling unacceptable unless you produce. Many people with ADD feel that they will not be accepted by others unless they work that hard. But this type of work ethic is not healthy, and it needs to not be anyone's goal. This is self-discipline as a response to living in fear. This is a very unhealthy way to live emotionally and usually results in depression and anxiety. Unconditional acceptance, so crucial for feelings of security and worth, is simply not present in the lives of people who are driven by this type of self-discipline.

If you recognize yourself in this description, it is time to take action. I want to encourage you to learn to play, to be creative in your own ways, and find environments that fit you appropriately. By doing that, no matter what your age, you can recover from crippling self-discipline and be a flexible, creative, relaxed, *and* disciplined person who will feel good about yourself.

Remember, none of us is acceptable to everyone—nor can we do everything. Just be yourself and exercise your own personal wonderful talents. You will attract and surround yourself with people who will support you and accept you *as you are*.

ORGANIZATION AND THINKING

Once you have a project, creative or otherwise, that fits, you have to have the organizational skills to pull it off. Even when you have a tremendous passion for your project, you must bring organizational skills to the mix in order to complete the project.

The trick is to use the form of *internal* organization that people who are ADD naturally have. Trying to apply linear organizational skills to your work usually won't work. Even if you work with a partner who is linear, you are going to tend to think in your own unique way, shaped by your ADD wiring. There is nothing wrong with that. It can be your strength if you let it. Use it.

To show you what I mean, I am going to the share with you the process I'm going through right now as I attempt to write this section.

I start off each chapter by speaking on the phone with my editor. We discuss the chapter—what I want to convey, which points are particularly important, how this chapter relates to others in the book, and so forth. From that phone conversation, she writes an outline for me. When I sit down to write each chapter, I use that outline as my guide. This system works very well for me. I am able to use my strengths, and I have help with the part that might be difficult for me—organizing my thoughts and material in a way that will be easiest for the reader to access.

When I began to write this section about the internal style of organization that is natural for people with ADD, this is what my outline said: "Lynn, I think this little section is going to be pretty hard to write because it deals with a topic that is going to be foreign to almost everyone reading it for the first time. I think an example would be helpful, but it should be a very short one without too many steps or connections."

As soon as I read those words, I felt a familiar twinge in my solar plexus. It's going to be pretty hard to write. Those words echoed in my mind. I thought, in a very linear fashion, Where am I going to get this example? How am I going to get across the point I want to get across?" I started to worry. I thought about my files filled with stories and the many people I've met who are ADD. I wondered if the *right* one would come forward in my mind.

Then I realized I was trying to *think* about the whole thing. But in situations like this, what I do best—and what so many others with ADD do best—is to *feel* about the whole thing. Not think, in the traditional sense, but feel.

It was then that a little light bulb went on in my mind. My head began to feel slightly light, as if it had expanded outward just a little. I instantly recognized that feeling. It's a physical experience I've learned to trust. It signals that an answer to my question is in the works.

Next I realized that I could solve the challenge of coming up with the example I needed by describing the organizational process that was happening at that moment. The answer seemed to be given to me as if magically. But it's not magic. Some part of my brain worked on solving the assignment. It wasn't the part of my brain I would call my "thinking mind." But it worked nevertheless. As usual, it presented the solution in whole form, rather than in pieces that I must string together.

How exciting! I felt joy throughout my body. My eyes were twinkling, at least from the inside, and I had a little smile on my face. I was eager to write and knew exactly what to write.

You put the question inside of yourself. You don't think. You stay aware and report on what happens. That's it! I can organize the production of anything that is creative that way. It always works for me. It can work for you, too.

People who are ADD and creative *are* organized. Information is organized in our brains. But it is organized differently than it is in the brain of someone who has more linear wiring. My internal organization is such that I think of things at the appropriate time. I never know ahead of time what I'll think up or what images I'll see. But they always come at exactly the right moment. I've learned to trust them and the little nudges and urges from within.

I cannot tell you how many times my editor and I arrive at the same image or the same way of structuring a chapter section at the same time. We've noticed this happening more and more as we work together, but we arrive at our ideas by totally different pathways.

For example, the material that is in this chapter, about organizational skills, was originally mapped out to be included as part of chapter 9, "Learning and

Creativity for the ADD Individual." But when we were discussing the material, I began to feel a feeling of discomfort. This uncomfortable feeling is one I associate with "something is wrong with this picture." I didn't initially know what was wrong, but I knew that something we were discussing just wasn't right.

We'd been discussing the teacher-learner relationship and how to protect yourself and build a partnership. As I *thought* about what I was feeling, I visually saw that relationship in my mind's eye as a center pole made of wood to hang things on. But I couldn't get organizational skills and other practical problems to both hang on that pole. They kept ending up somewhere else.

Meanwhile, my editor was thinking about the structure of the chapter and logically was coming to the same conclusion: a chapter about teacher-learner relationships was different from one in which I'm talking about developing organizational skills and self-discipline. Those topics needed to be in separate chapters.

Almost simultaneously we voiced the same issue. I said, "Something's wrong here. It has to do with practical problems versus having a teacher-learner relationship." My editor said, "I think we need to look at the outline for the chapter again and restructure it. I have some ideas how to do it."

We agreed immediately, explained our process to one another, and went through the steps of creating a new, separate chapter called Overcoming Practical Problems. We laughed and felt a wonderful warmth from the realization that we were so much in sync even though we are differently wired. We also instantly realized that we were living examples of the very issues that are faced by any two people with two very different ways of being wired. Each works, and each is fine.

Some of what I've come to realize is that my internal organization provides me with ideas, plans, and structure exactly when I need them—not ahead of time, but at appropriate times. I have to be *involved* directly with the project, though, rather than *thinking about* it for those ideas or plans to come to me. The sequence of thoughts and awarenesses happen spontaneously.

For example, when I'm giving a speech, I will ask who is in the audience and what they want to hear about. People speak up and ask questions. My mind instantly comes up with the first things to say in response, then the second that is tied to the first, then the third, and so on. In retrospect, there is often even a logical order to what I've said. But none of it was planned ahead of time.

This is part of the reason I love to be asked questions. A question cues a series of responses that even I learn from. I am much more verbally creative and interesting when analogies and stories pop into my mind *as I need them* than if I were to try to write or outline a speech three weeks in advance. Often, I've never even thought of the analogy or story before I speak about it. Fresh material appears when I need it.

Often one thought can lead to another in my mind, and sometimes even I don't recognize the connection between them at first. But the connection becomes apparent a little bit later. When it does, I realize that my mind was organized all along. It is just a type of organization that is different from the organization that comes when we *think* everything out in advance.

I've learned not to waste my time trying to solve certain problems the linear way. I just tell my mind what the question is and watch for an answer. I often do only one piece of a problem at a time, knowing that the next piece will come together when it is time for it to come together. From past experience I now have faith that this kind of organizational process will work for me. It always does. The only times I get lost and confused are when I try to solve a problem or create something in a linear way. I always end up tense and unsuccessful when I do.

But I have to play a part in this ADD type of organization, too. When people, materials, or ideas come to me that can be used to solve a creative problem, I'm very canny in recognizing that they are a part of the solution I'm looking for. I usually instantly recognize where they fit in the puzzle, and that's very important. If I don't recognize a piece of the solution when it comes to me, it could just slip by, and my problem would remain unsolved.

I recognize what fits, even if it's in a different language system. I recognize the offerings of my editor even though they come in a linear form. My mind seems to translate them to my system, and they end up as a feeling for me to experience.

So is this process that I'm describing the process of a *disordered* mind? Do I have a deficit? Well, in a way, yes. But I also have something that many others don't. Does the linear person have a creative/analog processing deficit? Often, yes. But that person doesn't have to carry a label of Creativity Deficit Disorder or Intuition Deficit Disorder.

Often people who are ADD can't articulate how they think or arrive at solutions. So some have bought into the party line that they are deficient, illogical, and off track. They have been separated from the natural way in which their minds can work. Reconnecting to the natural, feelings-style processing of an ADD mind will bring organization to anyone who is ADD. It's a system that has to be honored and respected, so it can be recognized by anyone who is ADD.

Sometimes people who are creative and ADD are accused of sitting around doing nothing rather than actively working on the solution to a problem. That may be how it appears to someone on the outside who doesn't understand, but that's not what's happening. If you are ADD, taking responsibility may mean asking yourself the question at hand or posing the job to be done, then putting the question in the back of your mind and allowing the answer to be generated. Meanwhile, you might just as well sweep the floor or play volleyball. Check in from time to time to see how the "fermentation process" is coming along. Allow time to bring the answers forward, and you'll finish the problem-solving part of your project. If I had not sat down today to write this chapter, it wouldn't have been written. But, once we carve out the time to do whatever it is we want to do, there's no use in forcing the answer prematurely. Let the process work.

That's how to be responsible when you're ADD.

Pay attention to your thoughts, to what happens around you, to the people and ideas that cross your path and recognize when they can be parts of the solution you are looking for. If you will follow your own way of organizing your work, you will find that your creativity will flow.

Truly the only times that I have had trouble being productive were when I was trying to use linear organization skills to accomplish tasks at hand. That's just not me. It might not be you, either.

The Linear Organizational Skills You Need

Now comes what I think of as the hard part. At certain parts of the creative process you may have to switch from your nonlinear organizational way of doing things to the use of linear organization skills. But because you are ADD, you may find that next to impossible. You also might begin to have trouble with the more linear issues of time management and keeping track of details.

If you are an artist, for example, you have to be able to find your materials and order new ones in a timely manner. You have to be sure that your environment is orderly enough to avoid accidents and messes that can ruin your work. If you're in business as an artist, you have to keep track of your expenses and billings if you want to *stay* in business. If you don't work in a creative business, then you must organize your time so that you can pursue your creative projects.

There are so many details to keep track of—phone numbers for networking, the cost of supplies and materials (for IRS reports), upgrades on equipment, warranties, money and checkbooks, information about your field, and so on.

Here are a few suggestions that may help you. Use what feels right, but don't feel you must do everything suggested. Ultimately, you must develop your own organizational system. No one says, though, that you can't enlist the help of others to develop it. Network with people who understand the ADD style of brain wiring, and you'll find your way.

Set deadlines for yourself.

Once you've decided upon an agenda, it's very useful to pull out a calendar and set some deadlines. They create a framework for you to hang your work on. Unlimited time causes too much room in which to roam around, continuing to create new ideas instead of following through on the one you've chosen to work on.

You may want to use a monthly calendar with boxes so you can see the whole month at a glance. Some people like to make or buy a big calendar that can be hung on the wall—one that hits you in the face every single day. Computer scheduling software is also available for people who like computers.

Be sure to schedule planning deadlines as well as time for internal processing of information. You might write, "Sit on the swing," or "Do nothing" so that you have the time to just germinate ideas.

Mark your final project deadline on your calendar, but never just leave it at that. Be sure to break the whole project into sections. For example, with this book, I marked the date I wanted each chapter completed. That way I could tell if I was running on time or ahead or behind. Since people with ADD tend to have trouble breaking long-term projects down into small bits, it's important to mechanically break them down so that we don't get lost between the start and finish of a project.

When you set up calendars or other organizational charts, you provide yourself with continuous visual cues that actually help train your mind in linear thinking. I'm not trying to change you into a linear person, but it is helpful to have some linear skills available to you—ones that you don't have to keep struggling with year after year. Using calendars not only cues your inner system to get to work, it gives you permission to cut time out of your schedule to work on other projects. It validates the importance of the creative project and releases the brain to go into creative mode.

But what if you don't meet one of your deadlines? It's not the end of the world. Just try to get back on schedule next time. The deadlines on your calendar nudge you to push a little harder or give you permission to take a day off without worrying that you'll get too far behind. They are valuable.

USE VISUAL AND AUDITORY CUES.

You will do better with projects if you give yourself visual and auditory cues. For example, stacks of trays or files that are color coded can give you a visual signal related to your work. I put things in a file folder while I'm working on them and then put the file in a stack tray that is coded with a colored dot. I do each project the same way so I always know which color means "completed," which one means "to be worked on," "needs information," or "ready to be edited." All outgoing mail goes to the same place by the front door. All incoming mail goes in the middle of dining room table to be sorted during work breaks. I never put anything away in a file drawer if I'm not finished working on it. If I did, I'd never think of it again. For me, it would be "out of sight, out of mind." I know I must keep what I'm currently working on within eyesight.

Making notes—notes you can easily see—is a great way of keeping track of things. Those beautifully colored sticky notes help a lot. They can be stuck to your computer, door jamb, bathroom mirrors, dashboard, or wherever you can't miss them. My son makes notes or lists on big pieces of posterboard and hangs them on his walls. That way as soon as he wakes up in the morning, he sees his schedule in BIG PRINT. It works for him.

Your cues may look messy to someone else, but that doesn't mean you're not organized. That is important for you to remember. Since you have responsibility to keep track of things, you get to decide how you want to do it.

The most difficult part of making visual cues for ourselves is carving out the time to make them. It's not much fun, and you'd probably rather be creating something new. But *do it anyway*. If you need to, schedule in a special time for organization and mark it on your calendar. You'll know that is your time to think about your schedule, get organized, and make your notes or lists.

I usually do my organizational work when I finish a chapter. It's a kind of break time for me. Or I do it when the sun comes in the windows and makes it difficult for me to work at the computer. That means that for about two hours every day I have time available to put things away, get things out and sorted and to make lists. To be sure, I don't do two hours' worth of organization every day. What a waste of precious time from my life! But I *can* use that time if I need it.

Since I spend a lot of my time now in creative pursuits, I spend more time than I used to organizing them. But if you only spend a small amount of your time pursuing your creative activities, you will only need to spend a proportionately small amount of time organizing your creative projects.

Auditory cues, such as a timer or buzzer, can also help you get your work done. They can act as your signal to start or stop what you are doing. Your clock-radio alarm or a wristwatch alarm can be set to go off when it's time for you to take a break, end a break, or pick up the kids after school.

NEGOTIATING

The ability to negotiate is critical to any projects you do, whether or not they are creative projects. Negotiating means making a transaction or trade with other people. It also means negotiating within ourselves. People who are ADD often have trouble negotiating because of the way our brain is wired.

Have you ever had difficulty shifting from one activity to another, getting started on a project or stopping once you've started? Are alternatives hard for you to come up with when you bump into a road block? Do you often feel like throwing a whole project aside because one thing went wrong?

I attribute these typical ADD difficulties to what I call the "on-off switch." It's as if the phonograph needle gets stuck in one place and can't move on. As an example, suppose you decide to make an authentic leather outfit to wear to a charity ball. But you can't find the color or type of leather you've seen in your mind. You've checked all over town, but it just isn't available.

People with ADD typically respond to this situation by becoming frantic and not knowing what to do. It is not unusual to spend energy complaining, feeling bad, and generally failing to let go of the image you had in your mind of how you want to look.

Because your "on-off switch" gets stuck, you probably won't think of substituting another outfit for this year and trying the leather one again next year. Chances are you decide to just not go to the ball because you can't wear the outfit you had in mind. Maybe you won't even be in the mood to go anymore—all because of a piece of fabric you had seen in your mind.

Unable to negotiate internally, you are stuck.

Much the same thing happens when it's hard for you to start a project and hard to stop one. You have to be really tough with yourself to counteract the lethargy that keeps you from achieving your dreams.

Negotiating outside yourself with others is a big part of being successful in any endeavor, including creative ones. But trading and working with others to get what you need—negotiating—is especially useful to creative people and those who are ADD.

Many people who are ADD have felt inadequate for so long that they never consider asking for help. The idea of making a trade seems ludicrous. "What could I possibly have to offer?" they ask themselves.

If you're stuck on the idea that you must do it all for yourself, you will not be able to reach out to others to make up for what you don't have. Your "on-off switch" can get stuck so that you don't even think about making trades. But you do have options. You just have to learn how to identify them and make them work for you.

Here are some suggestions to help you get started.

1. Acknowledge that you do get stuck and try to identify when it occurs. Does it happen when you are starting an activity? Stopping an activity? Trying to shift gears midway?

2. Commit to yourself that you want to change and can change.

3. Ask someone to help you. Having someone give you a reminder will help change the pattern of being stuck.

4. Make a pact with that person that you will practice starting and stopping an activity with a reminder from him. Discuss in advance what might be a reasonable amount of time to work on this particular project, so that his cues to start and stop working will be at reasonable times.

After some practice with your personal helper, you will be able to switch to mechanical devices such as an alarm. Then you will be able to follow their cues to start and stop your work.

Just remember that you always have options. Ask someone to help you identify some options the next time you get stuck. After having help establishing Plan B and Plan C, you will begin to get the hang of identifying options. Before you know it, you'll be able to come up with your own.

When learning how to negotiate with others, you'll need to master the process of making trades. Here are some suggestions for getting started.

1. Start by making a list of things you would like someone else to do for you.

2. Make a list of things you can do. (These will be used for trade.)

3. Next ask one person to do one thing that is on your list. Ask her which of several things on your list she'd be willing to trade you for. (For example, I give a loaf of fancy bread to the woman who reconciles my bank statement monthly. She enjoys its wonderful taste, and she doesn't mind working on my checkbook for me. I feel I come out on the good end of this deal, but she seems happy, too.)

Learning how to make trades is so important. It can really make the difference between achieving your goals and feeling like a failure. No one can do every single thing well. When you make a trade, you are giving the services you do have in exchange for the ones you need. It's really that simple.

I'm going to ask you right now to make a commitment to practice making trades for what you need. Will you do it?

LYING AND FAKING IT

Sadly, people with ADD often have learned to lie to others and to themselves to save face and avoid the shame of failure and feelings of inadequacy. Year after year of being unable to keep up with others—others who are no smarter but are wired in a way that fits our culture better—leads many people to "fake it" or to outright lie about what they are doing.

Even lying to yourself can be a problem. "This time, I'll finish what I've started. I'll meet my deadline." Unfortunately, when these commitments are made while lying on a couch, the odds are poor that they'll be met.

No one really thinks lying and faking it are good characteristics. But they become understandable behaviors when you consider how much it hurts to feel inadequate or like a shameful failure, and how often people with ADD have been faced with those feelings. Nevertheless, lying and faking are nonconstructive behaviors and, in the long run, will boomerang and hurt you big time.

Lying about commitments that you don't, or can't, follow through on is a common scenario among people with ADD. Maybe you committed to provide twenty paintings for an art show, but then you just can't seem to get them done. Sometimes the commitments aren't the least bit realistic. But when you want something so bad, you make them anyway—fooling yourself into thinking you can do it. The need to please is that strong.

Lying about the way in which you can do things is another problem area. For example, Joe might say, "Sure, I can put those screen doors up for you." But he fails to inset the hinges and leaves a gap for critters to walk in and out at will. Joe's not a bad guy. It's just that his desire to be successful and win people's approval is so strong that he says he can do anything that has to do with building—and he feels he can do it better than anyone else. In reality he hasn't cultivated the patience or skill to do quality work, even though he hungers to. If Joe really wants to be successful, he'll need to buckle down and start learning the details of his trade.

Maybe you take on projects that don't fit you. But after years of faking it, having to do things you never wanted to do, you can't tell the difference between faking it now and doing something that you might really want to do. You have no idea what really fits you, so you may go through life pretending to everyone who comes along about everything that's presented to you.

Even when you do pull off a job that way, you suffer from stress and strain. For example, when Trish was twenty-three, she took a job at a local recreation center teaching ceramics. The problem was that she'd never done any ceramics. But every afternoon before the class she'd go to a friend's house, learn a different technique for making pottery, and then go right to class to teach it.

Everything went fine until she had to fire the kiln. She had no idea how to do it. Her friend gave her some general instructions but they proved to be inadequate. Trish blew up almost everything in the kiln. Needless to say, that was the last time she tried to teach ceramics. In retrospect, twenty years later, she laughed about it. But at the time it was no laughing matter, and the price she paid was anxiety, stress, and strain.

Many highly successful ADD people have hidden feelings that they're faking life in general. No one else would know it by looking at them, but I'm here to tell you, those feelings are present.

Lying and faking it are patterns that can persist for many years until they feel like they're just a normal part of your life. But it doesn't have to be that way. Here are some suggestions for getting back on the road of truth and reality.

1. State out loud to yourself that you are willing to take the step of learning to tell the truth. It takes a real commitment to get started.

2. Next you must decide to attempt only what you are really willing to do and what fits you. That means you must be willing to say no to what you don't want to do and to what doesn't fit you.

3. Start small and say no the next time you are asked to do something that doesn't fit or that you don't want to do.

4. Congratulate yourself and realize that you are on the path to becoming an honest person with yourself and others.

To break the habit of faking it, you must be honest within yourself and learn to see yourself as a valuable person who does have skills and attributes that are valuable. To get started on that path, you can

1. Make a list of all the things you can do.

2. Make a list of what you like about yourself.

3. Have someone you trust—someone who thinks positively—also make a list of what you can do and what that person likes about you.

4. Study the lists. Put them somewhere in your home where you can see them daily.

5. Add to the lists regularly. (A support group is a wonderful way to find like-minded, supportive people who can help you.)

6. When you're tempted to fake it, refer to your lists and don't fake it. Say, "No, thank you. I'll pass."

When you're unsure about the quality of your work, consider talking with someone you trust and admire in the same field. You might want to ask that person how you could improve your work. That's a better approach than asking what is right or wrong with what you've done.

Remember, whatever the person says, it's only that person's opinion. Weigh it and decide whether you agree or disagree. But be open to learning without taking it to mean that you are an inadequate person. You can get into trouble when you mix up a need to better learn specific skills with a sense of personal inadequacy. Make the commitment to separate the two now. You need to unconditionally accept yourself as a wonderful, potentially skillful person who can learn anything you want to learn, as long as it fits you.

Just because you've been hurt many, many times by not being able to produce in an arena that didn't fit you, doesn't mean that you, the person, are inadequate. Once you really understand that, you'll be on your way to honestly being who you are meant to be—and feeling proud about yourself.

chaptereleven

Making A Living With Your Creativity

I F YOU'VE ALREADY won the lottery, or you've inherited so much money that your biggest problem is figuring out how to invest it, then you might not need to read this chapter. But if you're like the rest of us, you need to earn a living—and I want you to know you can do that using your creativity.

If you do want to earn your living using your creativity, you need to understand clearly that there are two parts to the issue: making money and utilizing your creativity. Earning your living with your creativity doesn't mean that you create what you want, when you want, and how you want and then try haphazardly to sell your creations. It means being committed to your creativity *and* to the issues that come with building a business. You don't have to enjoy the creative and business-building functions equally—and you can probably get help with the parts you enjoy the least. But if you want to make this work, you do have to be committed to both of them.

Let's start off by talking about the two ways in which people build careers: the internal approach and the external approach.

When you build your job or career based on what's inside of you, releasing and expressing your identity through your work, you are using the internal approach. You go within, on a feelings level, and find out what you're made of.

Or you study what you're made of, what you like to do, what you do naturally, and then make a career from it.

As you heighten your awareness about how you are really made, you will also notice how you naturally express yourself. You'll become aware of the environments in which you feel comfortable, and the ones you shine in, and you'll begin to see the many ways in which you express your talents and skills. You'll notice opportunities that come along, often at the very moment you need them.

You can think about this kind of approach as magical. But there really is nothing magical about it. It may seem so when people and resources suddenly appear that were never in your life before. You may notice others who have been there, but you didn't connect with them previously. But what's actually happening is that, because you have become alert to who you are and what you want, you are able to make use of everything and everyone who now crosses your path.

Sometimes the wonderful synchronisms that occur when you become clear in your mind about who you are and what you want seem to be spiritually guided. You certainly can look at them that way, but you don't have to. No matter how you explain it, the reality is that your newfound clarity about yourself and your desires and goals increases the likelihood that you will notice opportunities to help you accomplish those very goals.

An internal approach to career-building only means that you seek a job or career that fits you—one that you desire—and one that you discover because you know how you feel inside of yourself. You realize and value how you are made, including your ADD.

The external approach to building a career is based on strategic planning and thought about what job will benefit you. If you use the external approach, you expose yourself to a traditional set of opportunities in the job search—going to an employment agency, reading the want ads, checking with friends about what is open, and visiting with your college professors to discover what fields are hiring.

This approach also yields jobs, sometimes even jobs that fit your identity. But generally this job-board style does not fit a lot of people who are ADD. It involves a lot of detailed research and planning that frequently is not the strong suit of ADD people.

My friend Jean is a good example. She is interested in photography and computer graphics. When she moved to a big city, she began a job search by checking with employment agencies and checking job boards at the local market. She did find many leads, and she followed up on all of them. But, although she is a very good worker, she did not find anything that really interested her.

She felt she *should* get to work soon and almost took a job that seemed okay, at least from the standpoint of money. It wasn't exactly what she wanted to do, and her heart wasn't in it. But she wasn't sure what she would tell her family and friends if she didn't take the job. She really felt she had no choice. However, during her final meeting with her prospective employer, Jean's stomach twisted into knots, and her throat felt dry. She just couldn't get herself to say yes.

The next week, Jean heard about a job with less pay, but one in which she could be exposed to some of the computer software packages she wanted to learn about for her graphics work. She felt excited, figured her budget, and realized she could cover her expenses even though she wouldn't save as much as she had hoped.

As soon as she started the job, she felt hopeful that she would be able to build a creative career—one that she could eventually turn into self-employment, which is what she really wanted. Her heart told her she'd made the right choice. Her mind decided Jean had done the right thing for herself.

Making The Decision: To Use Your Creativity in Your Job or Not

You have a lot of choices to make if you are considering whether or not to use your creativity to earn your living.

If you're entering the job market for the first time, you can choose to look only for jobs in which you can use your creativity. If you're already in the job market, you can stay at your current job but try to introduce more creativity into your work. You can choose to leave your current job and look for one that would involve more creativity. Or, you can stay in your current job and keep your creative work separate, as more of a hobby.

Neither of these choices is inherently better than the others. The issue is what's best for you. What you choose for now may or may not be what you continue to do in the years to come. You have choices and can make choices as you change your mind. After all, you're in the driver's seat.

If you are just now entering the job market and you want to use your creativity to make a living, here's how to get started.

1. Assess your skills. You might want to do this by making a list of all the things you can do, including natural talents as well as learned skills. Believe me, there are many, many things you can do.

When you've finished your list, have someone, or several people, close to you go through it so they can add things you omitted. Then go back and put a plus sign (+) by the items on your list that especially please you and make you feel good. These are the talents or skills you are proud of and would like to use more. Put a minus sign (-) by any you would rather not do anymore. Then draw a circle around two or three of your talents or skills that you would *love* to use a lot. Those are the ones you would like to make into a career.

Then evaluate your talents and skills to see if they are strong enough to stand alone at this time. Do you need more experience before you commit to earning a living with them? Be honest here. For example, you might enjoy drawing and have some natural talent for it. But you might need a few more years working on your drawing skills before you try to get a job as an artist.

2. Do you want to work for yourself or someone else? You don't have to make a firm decision about this now. But if you do have a strong feeling about it immediately, one way or the other, go ahead and make the decision.

Some of the issues to consider are the freedom and responsibility you would have working for yourself, the skills needed to run a business, and money that is available to put into the business as a start-up. Ask yourself whether you can market and sell your work yourself. Do you want to? Can you fill orders and still be creative?

Again, if you do want to open your own business, ask yourself if you need to gain experience working with someone who owns a business similar to the one you're planning. I strongly advise it.

3. Gather business advice. You need to talk to an accountant or financial mentor, small business consultant or someone who can advise you about the process of doing business. Whether you want to or not, you have to think about taxes, sole proprietorships, local laws and professional rules, rent, copying, computers, and on and on and on. Depending upon the particular business you're planning, you must decide how much you're going to do for yourself and whether you need others to work for you.

For example, if you write books, you have to decide whether or not you want to buy and sell them yourself—whether you self-publish or have a publisher— ship them, market them, and more. If you make dolls, you have to decide whether you will man a booth at craft fairs throughout your region, pay someone to try to get the dolls in shops across the country, or take them yourself. No matter what your particular product is, these are the kinds of decisions you are going to have to make.

There is a lot more to owning your own business than meets the eye. If this is something you want to do, you have to realize that your love of your creative project just isn't enough. That passion for your work is never going to be enough to keep you in business. You also have to learn the business end of things or hire someone to do that work for you.

If you are not interested in starting your own business and are already working for someone else, there are three ways you can introduce more creativity into your life: 1) You can change to a job that will allow you to use your creativity in some way in your work. 2) You can decide that you will make that change at some specific time in the future, and you can begin taking steps toward that change. 3)

You can decide to stay put with your present job and introduce creativity into your life in ways other than in your job.

Creative Talent or Creative Lifestyle?

I mentioned earlier that there are two different ways to experience creativity: having a specific talent or living a creative lifestyle. You can make a living with either—or both.

If you are more interested in living a creative lifestyle than exercising one particular talent, you can consider changing your family's lifestyle—if they're willing to give that change a try. For example, you could go from a high-paced city life to a life in a rural area that has a lower cost of living, and a job that honors your creativity. But in order for this, or any, move to be a positive one, it's important to bring the whole family in on the decision.

A man I know, Mac, decided to make this kind of move. Mac was raised in a small Texas town but went to college in a large city. Although there were things about life in the city that he didn't really like, he could see a lot of positives and assumed he'd get used to the negatives. After college he married and started a family.

But eight years later Mac realized he never was really going to get used to it. He talked with his wife about how he would like to live. Rather than working as a social worker for an agency—where he had to go to the same job every day, follow the same schedule every week, and deal with the anonymity of city life—Mac dreamed of making a living by doing a variety of jobs. He could remodel homes and buildings, fix machines, do the set-up for campaigns and conferences, deliver newspapers, and generally do a wide variety of tasks. He felt he would have no problem providing for his family when he *created* his new life.

Mac's wife didn't mind the change. As a teacher, she knew she could get a job almost anywhere. She warmed to the idea that she wouldn't have to drive in rush-hour traffic anymore or stand in long lines. She, too, knew her husband's skills and believed he could make it just fine. She often said that he was the most inventive, creative person she'd ever met. Besides, she'd been worried that he was losing the relaxed, carefree demeanor she'd always loved in him.

They decided to move. Mac did great, and his wife discovered creativity she'd never known she had. Within two years she decided to start her own after-school arts-and-crafts program downtown and found she loved providing a creative environment for the kids.

On the other hand, there's Pat. Pat felt that the rural area in which she lived was stifling her creativity. As a clothing designer and entrepreneur, she needed both better access to resources found in the city and the stimulation of urban activity. She dreamed of having her own clothing shop, but the needs of the people in her community simply didn't match the style of her clothes or the volume of business she hoped to do.

So Pat approached her two children and explained the situation. They agreed that the time was right to move. Besides, they figured it sounded like a grand adventure. Needless to say, there was quite a bit of adjusting to be done once they got to the new setting, but one look at Pat's face after a day of activity put the matter to rest. Her insightful thirteen-year-old commented, "Mom, you've come alive here." Then, as an afterthought, he added "You're sure a lot less grouchy since we moved."

Pat's creativity continued to blossom into a full-fledged creative lifestyle with specialty parties marking holidays, decorations for her children's events, and costuming for her daughter's teams and associations. Even her son benefited when Pat came up with the prizes for his club's fund-raiser. It seemed as if everything Pat did became a creative act. She and her children felt much happier—as did Mac and his family.

Each had found their fit.

IDENTIFYING YOUR PRIORITIES IN CHOOSING A JOB

If you are a creative person, your first priority in choosing a job will be your need to be creative. I have come to the conclusion that to feel good about yourself— to feel mentally healthy and emotionally happy—you must use your creativity, if you are a creative person.

My years of experience as a mental-health counselor taught me that anyone who is ADD and creative, but is not honoring that creativity, will develop depression as a response to the lack of connection with their creativity. When a person is continuously trying to do things that don't fit, anxiety crops up. Fears, phobias, and other restrictive symptoms result from not living out who they naturally are. Many addictions, in part, serve as an attempt to cover the pain of loss.

To respect the importance creativity plays in your life, you must take a look at your value system. What do you value? What is your life all about? What do you want to leave behind? What is important to you? Where does your need to be creative fit into your value system? How important is that need to you relative to your many other needs and goals? Take some time to think and feel about these questions, and you will become clearer about what your next step must be.

But you also live in a world that requires you to have money. So the making of money has to be a real priority. It certainly may not be at the top of your list and you don't have to organize your whole life around the goal of getting lots of it, but it has to be a priority if you plan to remain an independent person. Certainly if you have any family members depending on you to provide for them, money is an issue. Even if someone else is the main money earner in your family, it's important for your self-esteem and self-sufficiency to make money-or, at least, be *able* to make money—on your own.

Don't forget the great feeling that comes from receiving remuneration for your creative productions. Though making money may not be a top priority, don't overlook the value of getting something in return for your creative work. And remember this: *Thinking and talking about money, and making it a priority is not selling out your creativity.* Try thinking about it as a foundation for your "child within" to have a healthier, happier life based on the innate value of his or her production. I am not saying you *have* to be paid for your creative work—your creative work has inherent value whether or not you are ever paid for it—but I do want you to think about it.

Don't assume that making a change to become more creative necessarily means a lower income level. I do not see it that way. I also cannot say with surety that it won't happen. But don't assume it will.

For example, let's look at Shelly. Shelly quit a good-paying job to pursue her interest in designing multimedia computer software for children. At first, finances were tight. But she soon hit it big with a line of in-school teaching tools. If she hadn't pursued her dream, she would never have made it big.

Troy quit a good-paying job at a large architectural firm to pursue his interest in designing and building getaway homes for vacationers. He had a good plan, but didn't factor in the competition that surfaced at the same time he was getting started. He overextended himself financially and ended up losing everything he had. Troy went back to work for someone else, at least temporarily.

Finally, Kitty chose to separate from the financial security promised by her husband and go it alone for a while to see whether or not she could make a living with her creativity. She had always dreamed of selling her creations, but so far all she heard was that she was "talented" and had "a nice hobby." That made her feel like her creativity wasn't important—and that she was being patronized.

Kitty found a storefront apartment and set up her shop in the front. In the back there was just enough room for a bed. The bathroom had a shower and barely enough room to turn around. There was no kitchen, but she managed to cook on the same hot plate she used to melt wax and cook dyes for her projects.

Her standard of living changed drastically, but after six months she found she was happier than she had ever been in her life. Poor, but happy! She was amazed at how often she could make trades for services she needed. Even getting her car fixed only meant cooking dinner for the mechanic at the local garage. Kitty discovered a world she'd not known existed—one based on people helping one another. No one had much money, but they survived and had fun.

Kitty couldn't imagine going back to the life she'd led before—when the expression of her creativity was last in line for her attention, and no one really took her seriously. In her new environment, she was an artist. Everyone knew it and, best of all, she knew it.

Most of us have heard stories of people who live in their cars for months, so they don't have to worry about paying the rent, in order to work on something creative. They put the completion of their work as the one and only priority. Such people might be at a time in life when they are willing to absolutely go for broke. They are willing to commit to their projects no matter what it takes. And they are willing to put all other priorities behind them.

If you're going to do that, you have to be extremely focused and believe in your project and yourself absolutely. Such focus does not fit living a creative lifestyle. It does not fit slowly urging several projects forward. For people who are ADD and very creative, it means some Highly Structured ADD will likely be present.

Not everyone chooses to put all their energy into their creativity. Not everyone is at the right stage and time in his life to do that. But you *can* decide at any time in your life that you do want to put your creativity first.

That's what Doreen did. She'd lived for a long time doing creative work after hours. She never actually thought of it as just a hobby, but she didn't make it her first priority either. When she came to middle age, tired of living a "normal" life, she decided she wanted to throw all her resources behind her creative work. So she moved to an isolated setting, sold a lot of what she had accumulated over the years, and mentally focused on her writing.

Facing the fear of scarcity was the first thing that Doreen had to work through. Though she had money in savings, she soon had a negative cash flow. For several years, she earned as much money as she needed to live and occasionally, especially the month or two before her royalty checks arrived, ran short and withdrew money from savings.

But she knew this couldn't keep up. Her fear of scarcity kicked in and she became very anxious. She couldn't bear the thought of giving up the expression of her creativity, but also realized she needed to *do something* to reverse the cash flow.

Though she never had to live in her car, Doreen did have to focus every bit of her attention on affirming her creative life. She meditated and used affirmative prayer that simply stated, "I will hold to my truth and my identity that chooses to express in a creative way. I fully affirm that reality and give thanks for the abundance that I am provided to express my talents." Doreen continues to write, slowly narrows the gap between income and outgo, and stays committed to living a creative life.

But this lifestyle is not for everyone. Doreen, like many others who go for broke, are at a stage in life when others are not dependent on them. Middle-agers with grown children and younger people who haven't yet started their families are frequently most available to put their creativity first—above everything else. People at other stages of life usually have less freedom to make that choice.

But still, there's a mental discipline that is required—along with a firmness of resolve, courage and desire—to put creativity first. Talking with many people who have done this, I've not found heroes or superhuman people. I've simply found people who cannot *not* create. Over and over I've heard, "I have to create. If I don't, I don't live. That's just how it is for me."

If your soul yearns to live with creativity as your first priority, I can assure you that your time will come. You don't need to force it, and you certainly don't need to prove anything to anyone—except maybe yourself. When the time is right, the resolve will be there. In the meantime, you may just need to draw upon your patience.

Identifying Your Family's Priorities

If you have a family, others with whom you are interdependent, you will need to talk with them if you are planning a major change in your life regarding your creativity. You are not going to them to ask for permission to do what you desire. Rather, think of talking with them to get their input so that their needs can be met, too. You are seeking to create a mutually beneficial lifestyle change that respects every member of your family, including yourself.

The best way I know to do this is by having one or a series of family meetings.

A family meeting means the whole family, except very young children who could create a distraction, comes together to talk. No television, eating, or telephone interruptions. Schedule the meeting at a time that will not interfere with any family member's prior commitments. Remember that the family meeting is not a time to argue, but rather to state one's views, acknowledge another's, and come to some resolution that honors everyone. There should be no winners or losers at the end of a family meeting.

Here are some general guidelines you can follow.

1. Do not interrupt the person speaking.

2. Each person gets a turn to speak.

3. Each person can take as much time as he needs to express his point of

view. (Time limits for speaking are not necessary unless someone in the group has trouble being reasonable and tends to talk compulsively.)

The person calling the meeting might start out as Dwayne did when he called his family together to talk about his job situation. His wife, two children, ages thirteen and fifteen, and his father, who lives with him, made a group of five. He opened the meeting by briefly explaining how he had been restless for some time in his current job.

Next he said he'd been working on a plan and was ready to share what he'd decided. Then he told each person the limits within which he could live. He *had* to do something to be more creative. The timing and the location from which he worked, at least for a time, were negotiable. Finally he said, "I want everyone's input."

He did not ask about whether his decision to do something with his creativity was a good idea. That was non-negotiable in his mind. He did ask each person, children included, to think about what was important to them, what they need-ed to make their life good for them. This included where the kids were to go to school, his wife's work setting, the amount of money they each felt was important to have, how that money was to be made, how to manage their involvement with friends, how they would feel about moving, and so forth.

Dwayne asked at this first meeting that they share their initial feelings about what he presented and to think about the rest of the issues. He asked how long they thought they would like to have to think about these issues before recon-vening for a second meeting. In later meetings, after everyone's feelings and thoughts were shared, they would begin to work out a plan together that would respect each person's needs and wants.

With this type of approach, all kinds of outcomes are possible. Dwayne might decide to work out of his house and have his family stay just where they are. They might move to another locale. His daughter might spend her senior year of high school with a grandparent or friend while the rest of the family moved. His father might decide to underwrite the cost of moving the family or he might decide to move in with a friend. Any and every choice is possible including locale, style of living, and timing.

When my own children were nine and eleven, I had just such a family meet-ing. I wanted to write a book. I knew that would mean that for about six months I would work two hours every evening after dinner. At the time I was making our living counseling during the day.

I asked the guys how they felt about this. It meant they would mostly be on their own for homework during this time. We'd still have dinner together and time right before bed, but we wouldn't have time to play together as we were accustomed to doing.

After telling them what was involved, we broke up the meeting to reconvene in two days. They came back and said to go for it. So I did. And I'll never forget the night I finished the book. We went out for dinner, manuscript in hand, to celebrate. As I prepared to pay the bill, my younger son, Mendel, came up to me and said, "Mom, I'm glad you wrote your book. Please don't write another one until we're grown up. We missed you."

I listened, I heard, and I didn't write another book until he went to college.

IDENTIFYING YOUR NEEDS RELATIVE TO YOUR STAGE IN LIFE

Depending upon where you are in your life cycle, you may find that it is easier or harder to make a change so that you can utilize your creativity. I want to share three people's stories with you so that you can experience the breadth of possibilities you may want to consider. No two families will make the same decisions, but the process you go through will be similar.

LaKeesha and her husband have two small children, two and four. They are both creative and would like to center their work life around their art. They decided this is the time to relocate, while the children are young. With kids not yet in school, they are free to go anywhere without disturbing their kids. They want to move to a community with good schools and other artists living nearby. They feel certain this is the time to establish a creative way of life for the entire family.

Walt's family has teenagers. He and his wife talked about wanting to do something different. They, too, are a creative couple who believe they can make a living with their art. But each of their children is very involved with a group of close friends and activities at the high school. They decided to wait until the children graduate before making any major lifestyle changes. In the meantime, Walt and his wife are doing what they can creatively in off hours, while making plans for a time when they will be able to do their creative work full time.

Jacob and Gretchen are an older couple who have worked very hard for years. Poor as children, they value money and have been saving a lot so they can leave their three children each a sizable inheritance. When Gretchen became ill, though, they began to rethink their priorities. Their grown children joined in and made it clear that they wanted their parents to enjoy their life, not sacrifice for them.

As Gretchen recovered, she and Jacob talked a lot about their dreams and what they hadn't done with their lives so far. They discovered that they shared a dream of doing something creative-and they wanted to do it together. So they used Gretchen's healing time to make plans to shift gears and make a new life for themselves. They decided to take some of their savings and invest in a business that they would run: one in which their creative talents could flourish. They were very happy with that decision, and so were their children.

IDENTIFYING THE ISSUES: SHOULD YOU MAKE A CHANGE?

I'd like to sum up the issue of making a change—a job change to allow you to better use your creativity—by providing you with a checklist that may help guide your thinking. Think about each of these questions carefully. It's important that you answer them honestly.

Are you desperately depressed about or bored by what you do for a living?   ☐ yes   ☐ no

Do you dream of being more creatively expressive than you are able to be now? ☐ yes   ☐ no

What are your top priorities in your life? _____

Do you have some ideas and dreams of what you'd like to do creatively? ☐ yes   ☐ no

Do you want to make a living with your creativity? ☐ yes   ☐ no

Can you become more creative in the job you have now? ☐ yes   ☐ no

Are you at a time in life when you could make a change? ☐ yes   ☐ no

How much money do you need—really need—to live on? $ _____

Who will be affected by any changes you make?_____

How involved are your family members in their own activities that would be disrupted by your making a change? ☐ A lot   ☐ Some   ☐ A little

WHAT HAPPENS IF YOU DON'T MAKE ANY CHANGE?

If you feel that you just can't make a change now, you will pay the price in one way or another. It's difficult to know exactly how you will feel, but here's a checklist to identify what you might be up against.

Will you feel cheated? ☐ yes ☐ no

Does the thought of not making a change make you feel depressed?
☐ yes ☐ no

What price do you feel you'll pay if you can't make a change now? _____

Are you susceptible to using alcohol or drugs to numb your
disappointment? ☐ yes ☐ no

Are you argumentative when you are not creating? ☐ yes ☐ no

Can you introduce more creativity into your after-work hours?
☐ yes ☐ no

Can you develop a long-term plan that will give you hope that you will one
day be able to express your creativity fully? ☐ yes ☐ no

Whatever your situation, I would strongly recommend that you do not leave yourself in depression, set yourself up for addictive behavior, or settle for feeling anxious or being argumentative. Make a future plan instead. Search for small ways to be who you *really* are.

You may not have as much of an option as you think. If the result of not honoring your creativity is to feel miserable, or if you've developed emotional or behavioral symptoms, then you *have* to take responsibility for incorporating creativity into your life. I've seen far too many people who have put money and status above creative expression only to spend a lot of time getting counseling for the symptoms that resulted from that decision. Turning to chemicals, alcohol, or pills is also no answer. Underneath many chemical-dependency problems you will find a creative person who desperately needs outlets, but who has never been able to give himself permission to express who he really is. If this scenario sounds familiar to you, please take the time now to reconsider you priorities.

SELF-EMPLOYMENT: MYTH VS. REALITY

If you do want to make a career change in order to use your creativity, you have several choices. Self-employment is one choice that comes to mind for many people.

Self-employment sounds great, doesn't it? You envision yourself without a boss making your life miserable, with customers who are loyal to your business, with plenty of time to do your creative work, and with plenty of money coming in. I'll admit that it sounds pretty great. But the reality of self-employment can be quite different. I'm not trying to discourage you from considering it. But you do need to think it through very carefully and realistically.

If you are considering self-employment, this is the real question you need to ask yourself: What can you sell to make money?

I hate to have to say that many of us who are ADD don't put much thought into this question. We crave the feeling of not having someone telling us what to do. We really want to have creative power over our work. We may have plenty of ideas, and often hear ourselves saying, "Now *that* would make a great business," or "I bet that idea will make a million." *But,* can you make enough money to make the business worthwhile—enough money to live on?

I hate to admit how many times I've failed to ask myself this question. I have tended to jump right in and only later realize that there's a lot more to running a business successfully than one great idea. At times I've managed to fairly success-fully pull off the business. But other times I've lost my shirt, so to speak. There's not a whole lot of difference that I am aware of between the two experiences.

Recently, a friend of mine who's a lot more linear than I am began to think about starting a business. Her first thought was to do a needs assessment of the market to determine whether a need exists for the kind of business she's consid-ering. She wanted to know what kind of bottom-line money can be made from a well-run enterprise such as the one she is considering.

Knowing my friend, I realize that she will go about the design and imple-mentation of the business in a creative way. She is one of those people who truly lives a creative lifestyle. But she also has a large linear part to her that makes her creatively *successful* in business. I call her a "bridge person," because she has, within herself, both creative and strategic-planning capability. I'm glad she's my friend so I can draw on her skills.

In order to successfully go into business for yourself, you must have some prod-uct or service that people will pay you for. Even though there are a lot of other business issues that have to be worked out in order for you to be successful—issues that can be tough for people who are ADD—you always have to start out by ask-ing yourself what you have to sell.

Again, I would caution you to learn from my experience. One of my problems has been that I am often way ahead of my time. I try to sell something that the public is not ready for. If you, too, are a creative visionary, be forewarned. Starting a business based on what you believe or feel others need to make their life better does not necessarily mean that people are ready for what you have to offer. They may not want it. It may take years before they do.

Needless to say, it has rarely occurred to me to systematically design a plan to create a market for what I have to offer. I'm usually way too involved with the cre-ation of the product/service/idea.

There are many paths you can take to determine what you have to sell. I'd like to share an example that both highlights the breadth of creative products and the kind of personal difficulty faced by someone who wants to be self-employed to sell a creative product.

My friend Dale has worked in computer science for twenty years. He has a driving need to be involved in more creative and challenging projects. What he really wants to do is work in the creative areas of robotics and artificial intelligence. That's what makes his heart quicken and his spirit soar.

Dale worked hard for several years to keep his money-earning job while starting a new business on the side—his dream job in which he would be self-employed. Even so, he eventually began to suffer mentally and emotionally and began to feel depressed because he couldn't do what fits him and what would make him feel good about himself. He was becoming fatigued and depressed from working two jobs: his day job that paid the mortgage and his after-hours work on his own projects.

Finally, Dale took the leap and quit his job to start his own business.

He loved it. He loved the creativity and the challenge and he felt great about himself. When I asked his wife how things were going, she said, "I feel happy, the kids are happy, and we're all happy and feeling great about ourselves." Dale knows how to solve problems as they arise, and that bodes well for his success. It's part of what goes into making a success—resilience and the ability to solve problems when they come up. And they always come up.

Some people, like Dale, have strong skills in this area, and others don't. Know yourself, and factor all your strengths and weaknesses into your decision about whether or not to become self-employed.

Self-Employment: Should You Give It a Try?

To help you evaluate whether self-employment is for you, consider the following elements.

Do you have an idea for a business? Is there something you love to do creatively that you could turn into a business?

Here is a partial list of what people can make or do to support themselves. The list is actually infinitely long, but these are a few ideas to get you started: software development, desktop publishing, computer graphics, writing, making jewelry, woodworking, ceramics, landscaping, handyman work, traditional crafts, traditional arts, teaching classes on almost any topic, baking, catering, opening a restaurant, raising plants or animals for sale, construction work, advertising, consulting to any company or person about anything that you know more about than the average person, providing training in an area in which you have experience and contacts. Now you take over and name several dozen more.

Here are some examples of jobs that weren't even in existence until someone took their creative passion and asked themselves how they could turn it into a money-making job: taking animals to visit nursing-home residents, being personal shoppers, maintaining indoor plants for businesses, and mobile pet-grooming. Can you name ten more?

For some people the creative passion is in building a business itself. For others, the creative passion is solving business problems as they come up. The list is endless and is limited only by the limitations of one's creativity.

If you're considering going into business for yourself, and you know you have the passion and commitment that it takes, then you need to make sure you have the right tools. I don't just mean mechanical tools, though those are also important. I mean the people support and networking that you'll need, to fill in where your own limitations surface.

For example, if you are a writer you need more than just a good idea for a book. You might need a computer with a modem and maybe an online service, a telephone with an answering machine, a fax machine, and the ability to easily and inexpensively make duplicate copies of your work. You may also need an agent, an accountant, a trustworthy editor, and a general business consultant. And don't forget a cheerleading squad.

Consider the mix of people you desire on your team. Though you are the creative force behind the business and are ultimately responsible for its success or failure, you cannot do it alone. Reach out to others who can help you.

Be realistic about how much and what kind of help you need for planning, marketing, sales, accounting, financial projects, inventory, and so forth. Just because you have a talent doesn't mean you can earn a living being self-employed and using that talent. But just because you are deficient in many of these business requirements doesn't mean you *can't* be self-employed. Choose your team members well.

The truth is that those of us who opt for self-employment usually don't think a whole lot about the choice. We often feel generally unemployable—creative, ADD people can be quite opinionated, with a need to do our thing in our own way. We live from the heart and *have* to utilize our creative nature, even if it means bumping and bouncing along for a while to get a business off the ground.

All I can personally say is "thanks" to all the people who have helped me— even the ones who, at face value, have done me in. I've chosen to learn from every step I've taken. Some have been hard lessons, but I try not to repeat the obvious mistakes too often. I continue to upgrade the skill level of the people I ask to join me. I sure have learned to let go of those who talk more than they pro-duce—and to do it quickly.

CREATIVELY WORKING FOR OTHERS

Remember, it's neither better nor worse to decide that self-employment is not for you. The image of the rugged entrepreneur who braves the cold snows for his art is basically an illusion created by someone who loves dramatics and wants to for-get the pain involved. Business, self-employed or other-employed, is just plain hard work on some days, good on others, and occasionally great.

If you prefer not to be self-employed, for whatever reason, find out whether your present employer is interested in using your creativity as part of your job. But before you go to your boss to discuss your creativity, take some time to think about the needs of your company from your boss's point of view. It's up to you to do that work. You're a lot more likely to get something that you will like and that will suit you if you've done the legwork.

Once you figure out what your company's bottom-line needs are, use your cre-ative talents to solve the problem, and you may come up with a deal for yourself. How different from going in and whining, "I'm bored with my job. I need some-thing more creative to do," then sitting down waiting for your boss to come up with something.

You may also want to consider switching jobs. Try networking to learn about jobs that would use your creativity. Be sure you have a clear picture of what you have to offer, and always keep the needs of any company or business in mind. Do a needs-assessment first. Then make an offer to solve their problems. That's always the best way to work it.

You can also try employment agencies or career counselors, but most don't work particularly well with people trying to find creative, unique jobs. What we really need to have is networking within the ADD community, perhaps through ADD organizations, for creative job opportunities. Now there's a creative job for someone to develop! Start your own creative job counseling business helping ADD people prepare for seeking work using their creative talents. Consult with companies to create ADD-friendly, creative jobs. Do workshops on how to cre-ate-a-job for yourself.

Of course it's not just people with ADD who could use creative job counsel-ing. Everyone would benefit from having their creativity tapped. I'd like to share a personal example that demonstrates this.

As I've mentioned, my work and my well-being have been greatly enhanced by the addition of my "personal editor" to my life. In reflecting about how it happened, I realize that not only was the expression of my creativity enhanced, but my editor's creativity was tapped by a third individual who worked in a very creative way. The story goes like this.

My agent, Mary, and I were talking about my writing and my desire to make the transition from primarily being a counselor to a writer. The problem was that it took me a long time to structure a book—a very ponderous, long time. I wrote all over the place, with millions of words and ideas rather chaotically floating around in my mind and on paper. The material and ideas were good, but they needed structure.

So Mary put her thinking cap on—something that she does particularly well—and came up with the suggestion that I find someone who could build an outline from my ideas, an outline that I would then write from. She asked me if I knew anyone who might be able to do that. I thought about the writers who had interviewed me for newspapers and magazines.

One in particular stood out in my mind. I remember that I'd felt my ideas were especially well reflected by Janis, a writer I had worked with recently. I had really enjoyed the interview with her and, upon reading the finished article, felt she had truly captured what I had said.

Mary suggested I call her to see if she would consider taking on the job of outline construction. Janis said she had never done that before and didn't have any experience with book writing. She wasn't sure if she could or wanted to do this kind of work, but she consented to talk with Mary.

Mary, in turn, saw potential that, at the time, Janis wasn't aware of. A bit nervous, Janis agreed to give it a try. We worked together on the first two chapters of the first book we were to collaborate on. It was slow going at first, but soon Janis suggested a way to speed things up, and we found the groove we've stayed with ever since. What a marvelous team we've made! I feel Mary opened a world of possibilities to me. Janis feels that Mary came along and released Janis's talents. For both of us, Mary's creative problem-solving and networking have paid off wonderfully.

The irony is that I'm not sure that Mary would see herself as a creative person. But Janis and I do, and that's what counts.

DECIDING TO MAKE THE CHANGE SLOWLY

Perhaps you would be more comfortable opting to slowly make a transition to utilizing your creativity. Allow yourself to slowly change your focus and the priorities that shape your life. Let your thought processes and feelings gently shift.

Perhaps you simply hold the status quo financially and let some opportunities go on the money-making side to look for opportunities on the creative side. Maybe you start cutting back on your lifestyle and expenses to give yourself more freedom to concentrate on the creative side of things.

Callie's dream is to start her own school based on teaching through the creative arts. Rather than jumping in all at once, she has chosen to make a slow transition. In April she was given three job offers. She took the one that allowed her to spend some of her time at work developing the curriculum for her school. While preparing for her current classroom, she is able to simultaneously research and create curriculum that she can use for her own school. That's a win-win situation.

Meanwhile, getting off work at a set time, she is able to begin networking with people who can help her find the financing for her school as well as building her board of directors and professional advisory board. Her team has time to begin to think about ways to market her idea. Her family has time to get used to the idea and adapt to the changes it will make in their lives. If there's a delay in establishing the school, she still has a source of income she can fall back on.

If you are working on a project and it doesn't go anywhere, sometimes you have to be willing to table it for a while. Timing is everything. Just because what you're doing isn't working out right now doesn't necessarily mean its a bad idea. You may only need to wait awhile until the time is ripe. Timing is important in transitions, so don't try to force things.

While you're nurturing your creative ideas and plans, it's a good time to start thinking about how you handle money. Use this time to keep close track of your money. Double check how your money leaves your bank account, asking yourself if you're spending your money in ways that bring you closer to your goal.

Sometimes people spend money to assuage feelings of neediness or frustration. If you have a solid plan in mind that will feed your desire to live more creatively, you may find that you can omit spending on something that is off track and put that money aside toward your goal.

I'm not saying to never treat yourself. We all have to live with some flexibility, and we sometimes need to give ourselves frivolous or nurturing treats. Just think first—so you do what is in your best interest—and you won't be sorry later.

The goal during a transition is to feel good about yourself while you're going through it. Your financial choices will help you achieve this goal without leaving you drained. Using your brain to think, as well as your feelings to feel, will help you move through this time constructively.

IF YOU DECIDE TO NOT MAKE A CHANGE IN THE FORESEEABLE FUTURE

Choosing to keep things exactly the way they are in your life is a viable choice. You may have completely assessed your situation regarding creativity and work, and decided to leave things just the way they are. You may have decided that you don't want to hinge your creative expression on money making, but rather, bring creativity out in your life in other ways.

You may make this choice because you like your job—even though it is not particularly creative. You may make it simply because you don't want to worry about money matters or feel you have to create in order to pay the rent. Or maybe you are not at the stage of your life right now where you want to, or can, combine creativity and job. Whatever the reason, I encourage you to give yourself permission to do exactly what you want to do.

You can make time to enjoy your creativity after work. Many people make their living one way and *have* a rich creative life outside of work. You will *feel* what will work for you.

Even if you don't do anything creative for a while, your creativity will not die. Sometimes the stresses or demands of survival make creativity dive underground, but it's not gone, I promise you.

Two months, five years, or twenty-five years from now, your creativity will be waiting for you. It doesn't matter whether you nurture it along the way or not. Haven't we all heard stories of the elder who begins to paint when he is 80 or the retired professional who develops a whole new business concept at 66? How about the 70-year-old woman who took up tap dancing at 65 and now taps her way into the hearts of everyone who watches her at the Opera House in downtown Bastrop, Texas?

No, talent and creativity don't go away. They just sometimes take a while to germinate. All you have to remember is to be aware of what you're made of and what you need. Purposely make choices to live your life the way you want to and gather your courage to follow your heart. Everything else will work out.

chapter twelve

Affirming Creativity

HROUGHOUT THIS BOOK, I have talked a lot about people with ADD using feelings to create, organize, and solve problems. Feelings, in my mind, are felt in the heart and expressed from the heart. Our heart receives all kinds of experiences and relates those experiences to the people we are, what we know, and what we want. The rest of the body receives those messages and expresses them further through our actions, thoughts, and dreams.

I sometimes think of feelings as a kind of electricity that flows through a conduit to a receiving station. The receiving station is the heart. The conduit is the heart path.

By feeling through your heart and by listening to your feelings, you will find your creativity. Your feelings are your guidelines. That's how the ADD-style brain works. Your job is to give yourself permission to follow what those feelings say—to give yourself permission to follow your heart path.

You are given creative desires for a reason. You simply won't have feelings or desires that don't belong to you. If you're doing something that feels good, then that is an indication that you're on the right track for you. If you're doing something that feels bad, it's an indication that you're doing something that is not on the right track, at least not at this particular time.

Your creativity is part of the beauty that you've been given because you were *fortunate enough* to be wired in an ADD way. It's part of what it means to be yourself.

The talents you have been given were put in your hands for you to make the most of. A person who is not wired in the ADD style is also given much to do but has another way of processing information and of reaching goals—usually through thought rather than feelings. Of course, it's not that a linear person doesn't ever feel. Nor does it mean that an ADD person doesn't ever think. But the natural, strong pathways available to us because of the physiological make-up of our brain is the gift that each person is given. It is the basic way that we each are programmed, so we can make the most out of our potential.

Much of your frustration as an ADD person has come from trying to use a pathway to completion that isn't natural for you. But remember, you wouldn't have a desire to live creatively just to frustrate you. All you have to do is take responsibility to recognize and nurture those desires using the pathway with which you are provided.

FINDING RESPECT FOR YOUR CREATIVITY

We live in a culture that is very mental, competitive, and judgmental. Your job is to step outside that framework and see a new vision of yourself—one based on the innate way you are constructed—rather than trying to adapt to one that doesn't fit you. There are other cultures that favor the ADD-style of wiring. But we just don't happen to live in one right now.

What I'm asking you to do is to move into a whole new paradigm—a whole new way of looking at your world and your relationship to it.

For example, if you wanted a container to hold water, would you choose a sieve and then criticize it for being dysfunctional? You must learn to choose a new container—to put aside the container that didn't work for you and choose something new. Your new container, your new setting, will be one that works well and fits for a person with ADD wiring. Once you make that shift, others around you will be able to look at ADD in a new way, too. As you experience less frustration and more success, they will see those successful attributes of ADD.

Frankly, it has taken me a long time to make this shift. That's because I was so strongly programmed by the culture in which we live. But I have made that shift now, and what I experience is tremendous respect for people who are ADD and for the creativity that is our legacy.

When you allow yourself to make that paradigm shift from the linear world to a world of feelings, you allow your creativity to be your guide. Yes, you still have to be responsible for yourself. You have to pay the rent or mortgage, pay your bills and meet your basic needs. You still have the responsibility to work within the framework of our culture. But you don't need to go about this living and working in a way that doesn't fit you. You can come to the same results by honoring your creative way of being.

I ask you to step outside of the way in which you have been taught to believe things *should* be done. I ask you to stop evaluating outcomes by the process you use to reach them. I ask you to believe in yourself.

In a way this calls you to be even more responsible than perhaps you ever dreamed you could be. Using your heart path to achieve your goals means that you must follow through with *your* way of doing things. No more excuses.

You may need to reprogram how you view yourself, trading failure for success and inadequacy for adequacy. As you do, you will let your feelings lead you, followed by your thinking mind to wrap things up. In the end you will be a whole person who has personal self-respect.

I personally ask you to take your newfound self-image and its innate power—innate power because you are being who you were always meant to be—and serve as a model for someone else who is just learning to find out who he or she is.

I ask you to team with others whose innate balance leans toward being non-ADD. As you do, you will find the respect that comes when all people bridge differences through working together, feeling together, and learning to trust one another.

Enjoy the value you have. Appreciate the value of other people. Team up.

Together, we will make the world a much better place for everyone.

INDEX